The Medical Lives of History's Famous People

Authored By

William James Maloney
New York University College of Dentistry
345 First Avenue
New York
NY 10010
USA

CONTENTS

CHAPTERS

FOREWORD

I met Dr. William Maloney years ago when he contacted me about how my grandfather, Babe Ruth, really died. His sickness was written about many times and discussed in many circles ... and everyone was mistaken.

Dr. Maloney changed the history, for me, of the passing of Babe Ruth in 1948. We learned much about my grandfather with his struggle to fight his sickness.

In reading this latest eBook of Dr. Bill's, I found it intriguing to read about all the famous personalities and how they met their fate. Some may amaze you. There are some important messages on how these people dealt with what they were handed, the defining moment when you have to face your own mortality. It will give you pause for thought.

Dr. Bill, you told me you admired my grandfather, well, I admire you.

Ruthian regards,

Linda Ruth Tosetti

PREFACE

"I do not feel obliged to believe that the same God who has endowed us with sense, reason, and intellect has intended us to forgo their use."

-Galileo Galilei (1564-1642)

Many lessons can be learned from examining the medical lives of the famous people throughout history. First and foremost is that nobody is exempt from physical sufferings, pain, ailments and the eventual death which all humans experience equally regardless of one's fame or finances. Nobody escapes. As Shakespeare wrote in 'Hamlet', "To die: - to sleep: No more; and by a sleep to say we end the heart-ache and the thousand natural shocks that flesh is heir to, 'tis a consummation devoutly to be wished."

All individuals deal with challenges in life differently. Celebrities are no different. Some, like Babe Ruth, think about helping others through their very own suffering. Some, like President Franklin Roosevelt, become more in touch with the sufferings of others and actually become more successful because of their physical challenges. Others are like President Kennedy who thought he had to suffer in private while trying desperately to be the larger-than-life person that society wanted him to be.

Authors have also given us fictional characters which examine all too real issues which all of us face during the course of our life. Such is true with Shakespeare's Othello, Fitzgerald's Benjamin Button, and Dickens' Tiny Tim.

Rich or poor, famous or anonymous, ruler or subject, beloved or despised- we all share the same basic human experiences throughout our life's journey. Maybe the real lesson to be learned by the medical challenges of the famous is to stop and analyze how we face our own life's challenge.

ACKNOWLEDGEMENTS

Special thanks to Clancy Marion Maloney for her technical expertise.

"This would demand the qualities of youth: not a time of life but a stage of mind, a temper of the will, a quality of imagination, a predominance of courage over timidity, of the appetite for adventure over the love of ease."

-Robert Kennedy

Special thanks to Dr. Maura Maloney for her guidance and support.

"... mystery and danger- we dance out 'neath the stars' ancient light into the darkening trees- Oh, won't you, baby, be in my book of dreams."

-Bruce Springsteen from 'Book of Dreams'

"Don't let it end like this ... tell them I said something"

-last words of Pancho Villa (1877-1923)

CONFLICT OF INTEREST

The author confirms that this eBook content has no conflict of interest.

William James Maloney
New York University College of Dentistry
345 First Avenue
New York
NY 10010
USA
Tel: 646-530-1276;
E-mail: wjm10@nyu.edu

ABOUT THE AUTHOR

Dr. William James Maloney is presently a clinical associate professor and a clinical pedagogical coordinator at New York University College of Dentistry of which he is an alumnus. He is also a graduate of Siena College in Loudonville, NY. He is the author of over 205 professional publications which have included many of the most prestigious journals in the world. These include The Journal of Dental Research, The Journal of the American Dental Association, and The Journal of Periodontology. He also serves as a reviewer and on the editorial board of many scientific publications. Dr. Maloney has received numerous accolades throughout his career. These include the American College of Prosthodontist's Achievement Award and the American Dental Association's Certificate for Service in a Foreign Country and an award, as a faculty member, from the Student National Dental Association of NYU. He has also been elected a fellow of the Academy of Dentistry International, the New York Academy of Medicine, the Pierre Fauchard Academy, and the Royal Society of Medicine. He has made presentations at various venues including the National Baseball Hall of Fame in Cooperstown, NY and the United States Military Academy at West Point. Dr. Maloney's work has garnered international attention. His work was the subject of an article in Sporting News magazine and has been featured on NBC News, The Detroit Free Press, and The Seattle Times. He has also appeared in a documentary, Universal Babe, which premiered at The New York Times Building in November 2012. In addition, Dr. Maloney maintains a private practice in general dentistry in Westchester County, NY.

CHAPTER 1

Hutchinson-Gilford Progeria Syndrome as an Inspiration for F. Scott Fitzgerald's Fictional Character 'Benjamin Button'

Abstract: In 1886 Hutchinson-Gilford Progeria Syndrome (HGPS) first appeared in the medical literature. An individual with HGPS exhibits many physical characteristics and ailments which are usually associated with the elderly.

F. Scott Fitzgerald published, in 1921, a short story entitled 'The Curious Case of Benjamin Button.' The central character of this story is born as an elderly man. It is postulated that Fitzgerald based his character on a real-life individual with HGPS. More importantly, it is theorized that medicine and society has viewed, in the past, these individuals incorrectly. These individuals might actually be experiencing true physical aging in a very accelerated manner.

Keywords: Aging, atrophic skin, Benjamin Button, coxa valga, delayed tooth eruption, F. Scott Fitzgerald, farnesyltransferase inhibitors, genetics, Hutchinson-Gilford Progeria syndrome, hypertension, LMNA, mutation, progerin, prominent eyes, tipifarnib, transcription.

F. SCOTT FITZGERALD

F. Scott Fitzgerald accurately described his own life when he wrote "There are no second acts in American lives." In a span of twenty years Fitzgerald went from being the most highly-paid writer in the United States, with some of the greatest novels of the twentieth century to his credit, to dying at the age of 44 as an alcoholic believing himself to be a failed and broken man. He could not have imagined that he would one day be considered one of the finest writers of the century [1].

Francis Scott Key Fitzgerald was named after his second cousin who wrote 'The Star- Spangled Banner'- the national anthem of the United States. Fitzgerald was born on September 24, 1896 in St. Paul, Minnesota to a couple of Roman Catholic faith. His father, Edward, was from Maryland and manufactured wicker furniture in St. Paul and later moved the family to New York to work for the Procter & Gamble Company. Fitzgerald's mother, Mollie McQuillan, was the daughter of an

Irish immigrant who became very wealthy as a St. Paul wholesale grocer [2]. When Fitzgerald was 12 years-old, his father lost his job with the Procter & Gamble Company and the family moved back to Minnesota to live off of his mother's inheritance [3].

At the age of 15, Fitzgerald was sent by his parents to a prestigious Catholic preparatory school in New Jersey, the Newman School. It was at the Newman School that Fitzgerald met his destiny in the personage of Father Sigourney Fay who saw his literary talents and encouraged him to pursue his dreams [3].

He later, at age 21, submitted his first novel for publication to Charles Scribner's Sons. It was rejected [4].

In 1917 Fitzgerald joined the army as a second lieutenant. He rapidly wrote his second novel entitled "The Romantic Egoist". Again, he submitted it to Charles Scribner's Sons. It was also rejected [2].

Fitzgerald was subsequently assigned to Camp Sheridan near Montgomery, Alabama where he became engaged to eighteen-year-old Zelda Sayre. He revised "The Romantic Egoist" and resubmitted it to Scribner's who, in turn, rejected it a second time. Upon the rejection of Fitzgerald's novel Zelda broke their engagement [2].

Undeterred, Fitzgerald set about rewriting his novel for the third time. He retitled it "This Side of Paradise" and it was accepted by Scribner's [4] and published on March 26, 1920 [2]. Suddenly, the struggling and destitute Fitzgerald was both rich and famous. He married Zelda the week after the novel was published. Zelda became a free-spirited individual who provided much inspiration for Fitzgerald's work. He often quoted her letters verbatim.

In the autumn of 1922 the couple and their infant daughter, Scottie, moved to Great Neck, New York to be near New York City as Fitzgerald's new play, The Vegetable, was about to debut on the Broadway stage. Fitzgerald thought he would make a fortune from the play. Unfortunately for Fitzgerald, Broadway theater was, and still is, very unpredictable. He was forced to write short stories to pay off the debt incurred by the play and turned to alcohol on a very regular basis

[2]. They eventually moved to Valescure, France in 1924 where Fitzgerald wrote his masterpiece, "The Great Gatsby".

At the age of 27, Zelda decided to pursue her dream of becoming a professional ballerina. She took lessons in Paris eight hours per day. Her health was damaged from three years of intense instruction. This led to her first mental episode [4].

Fitzgerald would spend most of the 1920's writing magazine stories as Zelda's mental health continued to decline. She entered the Johns Hopkins Hospital in Baltimore, Maryland in February of 1932. She would spend the rest of her sad life in and out of mental institutions. Fitzgerald would eventually fall in love with California movie columnist Sheilah Graham.

Fitzgerald suffered a heart attack and died on the floor of Graham's apartment on December 21, 1940. Zelda died a little over seven years later with eight other women trapped in a burning psychiatric hospital in Asheville, North Carolina.

At Fitzgerald's poorly attended funeral, the American satirist Dorothy Parker summed up his life by calling him "a poor son-of-a-bitch"- the same words spoken in "The Great Gatsby" at the funeral of Fitzgerald's most popular character Jay Gatsby.

'THE CURIOUS CASE OF BENJAMIN BUTTON'

F. Scott Fitzgerald published the short story 'The Curious Case of Benjamin Button' in 1921 [5]. The story is set in Fitzgeralds' father's native Baltimore, Maryland. It presents the case of an infant, Benjamin Button, who is born with the features of an elderly man. The infant is born as an elderly man and ages backwards. As time progresses Benjamin grows younger.

Fitzgerald provides many detailed descriptions of the physical characteristics and ailments of the central character.

He never names Button's disorder. However, the masters of literature have frequently used their incredible powers of observation of the human physical condition to find inspiration for their fictional characters. Literature is rich with characters who, at first glance, appear to possess the characteristics of some obvious product of the author's rich and vivid imagination. Rather, these characteristics are a product of the author's finely honed skill of observation. The author uses these observations to create a fictional character with the signs and symptoms of a real-life disorder. Many times these disorders are extremely rare. Some examples are the Grimm brothers' Rapunzel Syndrome, Oscar Wilde's Dorian Gray Syndrome, the Mowgli Syndrome from Rudyard Kipling, and Shakespeare's Othello Syndrome.

It is obvious that Fitzgerald was among these authors who used the physical conditions of individuals he encountered in his life for literary inspiration. He would take the actual written words of his own schizophrenic wife, Zelda, and put them into the mouths of his fictional characters.

I believe that Fitzgerald encountered, in his vast travels, an individual with Hutchinson- Gilford progeria syndrome and, in such an encounter, found inspiration for the fictional Benjamin Button. It is Fitzgerald's masterful attempt to interweave a documented medical abnormality into a fictional story.

The story begins in a hospital in which Benjamin Button's father is frantically attempting to find his newborn son. The doctor and various members of the hospital staff have already alerted him to the fact that there is something extremely unusual about the infant. Mr. Button thinks he is either insane or a victim of a cruel hoax as a nurse shows him his son for the first time. The nurse assures him that he is neither insane nor the victim of a cruel joke. Mr. Button describes the infant as resembling a man of approximately 70 years of age.

HUTCHINSON-GILFORD PROGERIA SYNDROME

There are many physical traits of Hutchinson-Gilford progeria syndrome (HGPS). Generally, infants with HGPS appear normal at birth and it is not until the first or second year of life that typical manifestations develop and become apparent [6]. Children then begin to display physical characteristics which are usually associated with those seen in elderly individuals [7]. The general physical characteristics include aged-looking skin, conspicuous veins running through the head, coxa valga, short stature, alopecia, easy bruising, craniofacial disproportion, high-pitched voice, micrognathia, horse-riding stance, dystropic nails, skeletal hypoplasia and dysplasia, decreased sweating, beak- like nose, decreased subcutaneous fat, thin limbs with prominent stiff joints, atrophic skin, sclerodermoid lesions, delayed dentition, mottling hyper-pigmentation, prominent eyes, faint midfacial cyanosis, delayed closure of fontanelles and sutures, protruding ears with absence of earlobes, flared metaphyses, and hypoplastic nipples [8-18].

A consistent and predictable characteristic of Hutchinson-Gilford progeria syndrome is the individual's failure to grow [19] while their motor and mental development is normal [15]. All individuals with the syndrome appear so similar that they could all be mistaken for being siblings regardless of their differing ethnic backgrounds [12]. The average lifespan of an individual with Hutchinson-Gilford progeria syndrome is only 13 years [12].

The disorder affects one child in every 4 million [20] with males outnumbering females by a 1.5: 1 ratio. There is a marked non-negroid prevalence [12].

A change from glycine GGC to glycine GGT in codon 608 of the lamin A (LMNA) gene is the genetic cause of most cases of Hutchinson-Gilford progeria syndrome. This change activates a cryptic splice donor site to produce abnormal lamin A thus disrupting the nuclear membrane and altering transcription [21]. Lamins are the main architectural components of a cage-like structure called the lamina [22]. Strength and support for the inner nuclear membrane are provided by the lamina [22]. The mutant lamin A protein product is known as progerin [15] and results in a complex downstream organ system disruption [23]. The genetic trait for Hutchinson-Gilford progeria syndrome is not carried by either parent. Rather, the gene change is a chance occurrence affecting a single egg or sperm just prior to conception.

A diagnosis of Hutchinson-Gilford progeria syndrome is made based upon its signs and symptoms [24]. However, there are presently genetic tests available which look for LMNA mutations. These test are now available because of the discovery, in 2003, of the gene mutation [25-27]. Prior to 2003 some other conditions such as Wiedemann- Rautenstrauch and restrictive dermopathy were commonly misdiagnosed as being Hutchinson-Gilford progeria syndrome [15]. Laboratory data from individuals with Hutchinson-Gilford progeria syndrome show increase urinary excretion of hyaluronic acid and elevated cholesterol or phospholipid levels. In one study 15 individuals with a diagnosis of Hutchinson-Gilford progeria syndrome were examined. All 15 individuals were heterozygous for the G608G mutation in LMNA [21].

The cause of death is primarily cardiovascular abnormalities [24]. These persons usually exhibit rapidly progressive arteriosclerosis [28]. Hypertension, transient ischemic attacks, and strokes usually precede death [15]. Other common cardiovascular involvements can be seen in the form of extensive atheromas, myocardial fibrosis, lipofuscin deposition, and strokes [29, 30]. Some CNS findings include vascular sclerosis with multiple ischemic infarctions, cerebral atrophy, and vascular myelopathy [31-33].

THE POTENTIAL BENEFITS OF HUTCHINSON-GILFORD PROGERIA SYNDROME RESEARCH

Since Drs. Hutchinson and Gilford first described HGPS in the nineteenth century very little scientific research has been performed. Fortunately, there seems to be a change in that trend. In September of 2012 it was announced that there has been a first-ever treatment for Hutchinson-Gilford progeria syndrome. This could potentially have tremendous implications.

Research will show us that Hutchinson-Gilford progeria syndrome just might be nature's way of presenting to us a rare and most precious opportunity to see the effects of aging in a dramatically accelerated fashion and, in so doing, allow us to understand the cellular and genetic mysteries of natural aging more fully.

REFERENCES

[1]   IMDb. F. Scott Fitzgerald. Accessed on 8/20/12. Available at: www.imdb.com/name/
       nm0280234/.
[2]   University of South Carolina. A Brief Life of Fitzgerald. Accessed on 8/14/12. Available
       at: www.sc.edu/fitzgerald/biography.html.

[3]   Bio. F. Scott Fitzgerald. Accessed on 8/19/12. Available at: www.biography.com/people/f.scott-fitzgerald-9296261.

[4]   PBS. F. Scott Fitzgerald and the American dream. Accessed on 8/12/12. Available at: www.pbs.org/kteh/amstorytellers/bios.html.

[5]   Fitzgerald FS. Flappers and philosophers: short stories. New York: Scribner's. Republished in New York: Cambridge UP, 2000.

[6]   Wisuthsarewong W, Viravan S. Hutchinson-Gilford progeria syndrome. J Med Assoc Thai 1999; 82: 96-102.

[7]   Progeria Research Foundation. About progeria. Accessed on 7/30/09. Available at: www.progeriaresearch.org/about_progeria.html.

[8]   Hutchinson J. Congenital absence of hair and mammary glands with atrophic condition of the skin and its appendages in a boy whose mother had been almost totally bald from alopecia areata from the age of six. Mediochir Trans 69: 473-477.

[9]   Manschot WA. A case of progeroanism (progeria of Gilford). Acta Paediatr 1950; 39: 158-164.

[10]   Thomson J, Forfar JO. Progeria (Hutchinson-Gilford syndrome): report of a case and review of the literature. Arch Dis Child 1950; 25: 224-234.

[11]   Warner HR. Research of Hutchinson-Gilford progeria syndrome. J Gerontol A Biol Sci Med Sci 2008; 63: 775-776.

[12]   Progeria Research Foundation. About progeria. Accessed on 7/28/11. Available at: www.progeriaresearch.org/about_progeria.htm.

[13]   Album MM, Hope JW. Progeria; report of a case. Oral Surg Oral Med Oral Pathol 1958; 11: 958-998.

[14]   Cooke JV. The rate of growth in progeria, with a report of two cases. J Pediatr 1953; 42: 26-37.

[15]   Csoka AB, Cao H, Sammak PJ, Constantinescu D, Schatten GP, Hegele RA. Novel lamin A/C gene (LMNA) mutations in atypical progeroid syndromes. J Med Genet 2004; 41: 304-308.

[16]   Fleischmaier R, Nedwich A. Progeria (Hutchinson-Gilford). Arch Dermatol 107: 253-258.

[17]   Ozonoff MB, Clemett AR. Progressive osteolysis in progeria. Am J Roentgenol RadiumTher Nucl Med 1967; 100: 75-79.

[18]   Gordon LB, McCarten KM, Giobbie-Hurder A, *et al*. Disease progression in Hutchinson-Gilford progeria syndrome: impact on growth and development. Pediatrics 2007; 120: 824-833.

[19]   Warner HR. Researcon Hutchinson-Gilford progeria syndrome. J Gerontol A Biol Sci Med Sci 2008; 63: 773-776.

[20]   Hampton T. Cancer drug and progeria. J Am Med Assoc 2005; 294: 2016.

[21]   Merideth MA, Gordon LB, Clauss S, *et al*. Phenotype and course of Hutchinson-Gilford progeria syndrome. New Eng J Med 2008; 358: 592-604.

[22]   Hutchinson CJ. Lamins: building blocks or regulators of gene expression? Nat Rev Mol Cell Biol 3: 848-858.

[23]   DeBusk FL. The Hutchinson-Gilford progeria syndrome. Report of 4 cases and review of the literature. J Pediatr 1972; 80: 697-724.

[24]   MayoClinic.com. Progeria 2012. Accessed on 8/16/12. Available at: www.mayoclinic.com/health/progeria/DS00936.

[25] Cao H, Hegele RA. LMNA is mutated in Hutchinson-Gilford progeria (MIM 176670) but not in Wiedemann-Rautenstrauch progeroid syndrome (MIM 264090). J Hum Genet 2003; 48: 271-274.

[26] De Sandre-Giovannoli A, Bernard R, Cau P, *et al*. Lamin A truncation in Hutchinson-Gilford progeria syndrome. Science 2003; 300: 2005.

[27] Eriksson M, Brown WT, Gordon JB, *et al*. Recurrent *de novo* point mutations in Lamin A cause Hutchinson-Gilford progeria syndrome. Nature 2003; 423: 293-298.

[28] Hennekam RC. Hutchinson-Gilford progeria syndrome; review of the phenotype. Am J Med Genet A 2006; 140: 2603-2624.

[29] Reichel W, Garcia-Runuel R. Pathologic findings in progeria: myocardial fibrosis and lipofuscin pigment. Am J Clin Pathol 1970; 53: 243-253.

[30] Baker PB, Baba N, Boesel CP. Cardiovascular abnormalities in progeria: case report and review of the literature. Arch Pathol Lab Med 105: 384-386.

[31] Haustein J, Pawlas U, Cervos-Navarro J. Homologous cerebral atrophy and ischemic insults in progeria adultorum. Zentralbl Allg Pathol 1989; 135: 51-56.

[32] Maloney WJ. Hutchinson-Gilford progeria syndrome: its presentation in F. Scott Fitzgerald's short story 'the curious case of Benjamin Button' and its oral manifestations. Journal of Dental Research 2009; 88(10): 873-876.

[33] Maloney W. The Integral role of the dentist in treating individuals with Hutchinson-Gilford progeria syndrome. WebmedCentral AGING, DENTISTRTY 2010; 1(7): WMC00446.

CHAPTER 2

The Extreme Darwinian Principles of Science Fiction Writer H.G. Wells Seen in Contrast to His Personal Views Concerning His Own Diabetes

Abstract: Diabetes is a disorder which affects millions of individuals worldwide. Diabetes refers to a group of metabolic disorders in which the body either does not produce enough insulin or the body does not respond to the insulin that is being produced.

H.G. Wells was well-known throughout the world for his writing in the science fiction genre. He also adhered to strict Darwinian principles. However, upon developing diabetes he became a staunch advocate for the access to insulin for all without regard for their ability to pay for it. Wells performed many noble and altruistic deeds on behalf of his fellow diabetics. This certainly did not correspond with his beliefs and attitudes in other areas of life.

Keywords: A1C, blood glucose, burning mouth syndrome, Charles Darwin, diabetes, gestational diabetes, gingivitis, insulin pump, ketoacidosis, pancreas, periodontitis, science fiction, tooth loss, Type 1 diabetes, Type 2 diabetes, urination.

H.G. WELLS AND DIABETES

Herbert George Wells was born on September 21, 1866 in Bromley, England. This individual would later become known to the world as H.G. Wells- the prolific author of many science fiction novels. These titles include 'The Time Machine', 'The Invisible Man' and 'The Island of Dr. Moreau'. On October 30, 1938 terror abounded on the east coast of The United States as a result of an adaptation of Wells' 'War of the Worlds'. In 'War of the Worlds' the reader is given a most enlightening glimpse of the disturbing social philosophies of H.G. Wells. In 'War of the Worlds' the weak are killed off and the Earth is again ruled by the strong (represented by the Martians) [1].

Wells was very influenced by the work of Charles Darwin. Wells became a strong advocate of the Marxist theories of class struggle. His science fiction was heavily influenced by notions and theories on society and eugenics. Wells became active in the world of radical politics believing in the possibility of a utopian society in which natural selection would play a large role in which the strong would rule and dominate over the weak [2] in a manner that could only be described in Wells' own words as being "with no pity and less benevolence".

In 1930 Wells was diagnosed with diabetes. At that time there was no distinction between the various types of diabetes. Today, Wells would be classified as being a Type II diabetic. Subsequent to his diagnosis, Wells' own desire to survive came to the forefront of both his personal actions and his socio-political agenda. According to the so-called logic of Wells' previous writings and public teachings it would follow that natural selection was placing himself on the wrong side of the distinct line he drew. Alas, he shunned those radical ideologies when it came to his own health and took advantage of the recently discovered miracle drug, insulin, to save his own life. Furthermore, Wells even had it somewhere in his heart to become an advocate and a champion of diabetics worldwide.

On February 15, 1934 Wells wrote an eloquent Letter to the Editor in The London Times [3] in which he brilliantly and accurately described diabetes as a rather simple disease to manage if the individual received the proper treatment. He stated that the diabetic is neither disabled physically nor morally and that the diabetic's thinking and intellect remains unimpaired. He calls for the creation of an association which would educate diabetics worldwide in the various aspects of the disorder and provide insulin to all regardless of their financial means. Wells went on to become a co-founder of what is known today as Diabetes UK. Wells lived until 1946, just one month short of his eightieth birthday. During this time his literary reputation diminished immensely mostly due to his continued radical attacks on various institutions and ideals.

H.G. Wells is known for his gripping science fiction. Wells had the ability to transport his readers into a futuristic place and time. Wells was also very progressive with his pioneering work in the field of diabetes education. He understood very well that a diabetic could live a long, joyful and complete life if the diabetic patient receives the proper education and nutrition. In addition, Wells knew that it is of vital importance for the diabetic to receive competent medical care and, if insulin-dependent, access to the life-sustaining drug.

Wells displayed kindred feelings of benevolence for his fellow diabetics. He needs to be remembered and lauded for this. Unfortunately, Wells' wonderful work for diabetics worldwide did not extend to any other aspect of his life. It certainly can be theorized that Wells was a hypocrite as he was a staunch advocate of eugenics and natural selection being applied to humans. The motive of Wells' interest in diabetes was obviously a selfish one. When confronted with a potentially life-threatening disorder, Wells quickly and, albeit intelligently, abandoned his ridiculous principles and sought the care of skilled healthcare professionals and the newly discovered miracle drug insulin.

DIABETES

There are three main types of diabetes. They are Type 1, Type 2, and gestational diabetes.

Some signs of diabetes include being very thirsty, frequent urination, weight loss, blurry vision, tingling or numbness in the hands or feet, extreme unexplained fatigue, increased hunger, irritability, wounds that do not heal, and frequent infections of the skin, gingiva or bladder [4] (Table **1**).

Table 1.   **Signs and Symptoms of Hyperglycemia**

-increased thirst
-high blood glucose
-high levels of sugar in urine
-frequent urination
-hunger
-headaches
-tiredness
-blurred vision
-difficulty concentrating

Type 1 diabetes is usually diagnosed in children or young adults whose beta cells of the pancreas no longer make insulin because they have been destroyed by an attack, for some reason, from their own immune system. It is treated by taking insulin [5].

Type 2 diabetes is the most common form of diabetes and can develop at any age. Physical inactivity and being overweight increases the chances of developing Type 2 diabetes [6].

Gestational diabetes may develop toward the end of pregnancy. It usually goes away after the child is born. However, a female who has had gestational diabetes is more likely to later develop Type 2 diabetes [6].

Today, a diabetic may replace the necessity of periodic daily injections by the use of an insulin pump. An insulin pump delivers rapid-acting insulin continuously through the use of a catheter [7]. There has been a dramatic increase in the use of insulin pump therapy or continuous subcutaneous insulin infusion in youths with Type 1 diabetes. There are both many advantages and disadvantages to insulin pump therapy. Some of the advantages include the following: 1) the elimination of insulin injections; 2) insulin pumps often improve A1C levels; 3) insulin pumps deliver insulin more accurately than injections; 4) it makes diabetes management easier; 5) results in fewer large swings in blood glucose levels; 6) allows flexibility regarding what food is eaten and when which improves the quality of life; 7) reduces severe low blood glucose episodes; 8) eliminates unpredictable effect of intermediate or long lasting insulin; 9) allows the diabetic to exercise without having to eat large amounts of carbohydrates [8] (Table **2**).

Table 2.   Signs and Symptoms of Hypoglycemia

-weakness
-trouble speaking
-trembling
-nervousness
-hunger
-sweating

Some of the disadvantages of insulin pump therapy include the following: 1) can cause weight gain; 2) can be expensive; 3) can cause diabetic ketoacidosis if catheter comes out and insulin is not provided to the individual for hours; 4) can be bothersome since individual is attached to the pump most of the time; 5) can require time in an outpatient facility or a hospital in order to be trained in its use [9].

Oral complications associated with diabetes include xerostomia, tooth loss, odontogenic abscesses, gingivitis, periodontitis, caries, soft tissue lesions of the tongue and oral mucosa [10-12] and burning mouth syndrome [11].

The most common oral complication of diabetes is the susceptibility to periodontal disease [12]. Individuals with poorly controlled diabetes are at a greater risk of developing periodontal disease [11]. Proper oral home care and regular dental examinations and cleanings are of paramount importance. Also, it is imperative that the negative periodontal effects of smoking be stressed to diabetics. Diabetics who smoke are 20 times more likely to develop periodontitis with loss of supporting bone structure than non-diabetic smokers [11, 13-15]. All diabetics should seek regular dental care. This fact is of extreme importance to the overall health of the diabetic individual.

REFERENCES

[1]   MacKenzie N, MacKenzie J. H.G. Wells: A Biography. New York: Simon and Schuster; p. 487.
[2]   Lawless G. The Harvard Crimson; The Evolution of H.G. Wells; accessed on 8/23/12. Available at: www.thecrimson.com/article/1973/12/14/the-evolution-of-hg-wells- pbthe/.
[3]   Diabetes UK. HG Wells's letter to 'The Times'; accessed on 9/19/12. Available at: http://www.diabetes.org.UK/About_us/Who_we_are/History?The-founding-of-Diabetes-UK/HG_weiss-letter-to-The-Times/.
[4]   Joslin Diabetes Center. General diabetes facts and information. Accessed on 12/26/12. Available at: http//www.joslin.org/info/ general_diabetes_facts_and_information.html? gclid=CKHOru67cuCFQ895QodQBZVmg.
[5]   U.S. Department of Health and Human Sevices. What diabetes is. Accessed on 3/27/12. Availablle at: http://diabetes.niddk.nih.gov/dm/pubs/type1and2/what.aspx#what.
[6]   Moore PA, Weyant RJ, Mongelluzzo MB, *et al*. Type 1 diabetes mellitus and oral health: assessment of periodontal disease. J Periodontol 1999; 70: 409-417.
[7]   American Dental Association. Insulin pumps. Accessed on 4/3/12. Available at: http:// www.diabetes.org/living-with-diabetes/treatment-and-care/medication/insulin- pumps.html.
[8]   American Diabetes Association. Advantages of using an insulin pump. Accessed on 10/5/12. Available at: http://www.diabetes.org/living-with-diabetes/treatment-and-care/ medication/insulin/advantages-of-using-an.html.
[9]   American Diabetes Association. Disadvantages of using an insulin pump. Accessed on 10/5/12. Available at: http://www.diabetes.org/living-with-diabetes/treatment-and- care/me dication/insulin/disadvantages-of-using-an.html.
[10]   Vernillo AT. Dental considerations for the treatment of patients with diabetes mellitus. J Am Dent Assoc 2003; 134(10): 245-335.

[11] Galili D, Mordechi F, Garfunkel AA. Oral and dental complications associated with diabetes and their treatment. Compendium Continuing Educ Dent 1984; 15: 496-508.

[12] May OA. Management of the diabetic dental patient. Quintessence Inter 1990; 21491-494.

[13] Glavind L, Lund B, Loe H. The relationship between periodontal state abd diabetes duration, insulin dosage and retinal changes. J Periodontol 1968; 39: 341-347.

[14] Shlossman M, Knowler WC, Pettitt DJ, Genco RJ. Type 2 diabetes mellitus and periodontal disease. JADA 1990; 121: 532-536.

[15] Moore PA, Weyant RJ, Mongelluzzo MB, *et al*. Type 1 diabetes mellitus and oral health: assessment of tooth loss and edentulism. J Public Health Dent 1998; 58(2): 135-142.

CHAPTER 3

The Historical Facts Concerning Babe Ruth's Heroic Battle with Nasopharyngeal Carcinoma

Abstract: George Herman "Babe" Ruth is remembered today as the greatest baseball player ever. Fans recall fondly his prodigious home runs and his many titles, records, and accolades earned on the playing field. In 1946 Ruth developed various symptoms in the head and neck region. He subsequently sought medical treatment and received a multitude of misdiagnoses.

Ruth had a relatively rare form of cancer known as nasopharyngeal carcinoma. To the present day, many misconceptions still persist surrounding his cancer. Today, we can truly view Ruth as a hero off the athletic fields for his humanitarian efforts in volunteering for experimental cancer treatments in order to help medical researchers gather very valuable information while fully knowing that such treatments would never cure his own cancer.

Keywords: Babe Ruth, baseball, Boston Red Sox, cancer research, cancer treatment, experimental drugs, Gate of Heaven Cemetery, Horner Syndrome, nasopharyngeal carcinoma, trismus.

GEORGE HERMAN 'BABE' RUTH

In every profession and walk of life there are individuals who come around but rarely and upon whom are bestowed such superlatives as giant, superstar, hero or some other superlative which attempts to separate the elite few from the rest of the pack.

Only one athlete is featured in this eBook for a reason. There have been numerous athletes who have been at the top of their particular sport and who have captured the attention and awe of a multitude of followers. However, in the case of George Herman 'Babe" Ruth there was and always will be only he at the top of the mountain.

The magnificent story of Babe Ruth takes us back to the dirty, squalid waterfront city of Baltimore, Maryland towards the close of the nineteenth century. On

February 6, 1895 George was born to Catherine Schamberger Ruth and George Ruth. Catherine would give birth to seven more children over the years but only George and his sister, Mary Margaret, would survive past infancy [1]. Mary Margaret Ruth would live to the age of 91 and be known as 'Mamie' throughout her life. This nickname was given to her by big brother George [2]. Some people called young George a trouble-making child or even a bad youngster but, as Mamie put it "he wasn't bad, he was only mischievous". The mischievous but good-hearted youth proved too much for his hard-working parents to manage. So, at the age of 7 George was brought to St. Mary's Industrial School for Boys. St. Mary's was only a few miles south of his family's Emory Street home in Baltimore. Sometimes on weekends Mamie would travel to St. Mary's with her mother to visit her big brother.

Almost miraculously, Br. Mathias, a physically-imposing man with a gentle heart of gold, became the mentor the child so desperately needed. The Xaverian brother and the young boy would form a friendship which would endure the rest of their lives. Br. Mathias would teach young George the game of which he was so fond-baseball.

Ruth enjoyed his years at St. Mary's. It would become very apparent during these years that George possessed a special talent for baseball. However, his days at St. Mary's certainly did not consist of only playing sports. George received a top quality education at St. Mary's. The penmanship taught to him would become obvious years later in his beautiful signature which is still coveted worldwide to this day. Ruth's penmanship was indicative of the discipline instilled in all the boys at St. Mary's.

Each boy at St. Mary's had to learn a trade. George was no exception. He sewed neckbands into shirts in a building adjacent to the baseball field. Sometimes George's shirt count was lower than it should have been and this puzzled the Brothers. George, always looking out for the smaller and younger boys or 'minims' as he called them, would make kites for the younger children. The kites would have long shirt tails on them. On cold days, George would convince the cook to make buns for the younger children. George would put warm molasses on the buns for the youngsters to enjoy [3]. Over the years George's physical talents continued to develop. At the age of 19, Jack Dunn, the top baseball scout of the time, signed George to a professional baseball contract. George's new teammates referred to him as 'Jack's newest babe'. George Herman Ruth now belonged to the people of the world simply as Babe Ruth.

Ruth would start his career with the Boston Red Sox as a pitcher and an outfielder. He was dominant at both positions. However, what attracted fans to the ballpark was Babe's incredible ability to hit home runs. This ability revolutionized the game and to say that Babe became a legend would be a huge understatement. Babe carried the Red Sox to three world championships and became beloved throughout New England. However, on December 26, 1919 Boston Red Sox owner Harry Frazee struck a deal with the New York Yankees. This deal would change sports forever and make Frazee the most despised man in New England well into the next century. The New York Times predicted that Ruth would break his own home run record the following year at the Polo Grounds in New York where the Yankees would be playing their home games [4]. The Polo Grounds belonged to another New York baseball team- the New York Giants. The Yankees would continue to play at the Polo Grounds through the 1922 season. Subsequently, the Yankees had to find their own ballpark as the Giants did not like the Yankees having larger attendance numbers than the Giants at the Polo Grounds. This was all because of one person- Ruth. Ruth had become a huge drawing card.

The following April Yankee Stadium opened. Ruth, never failing to deliver in the spotlight, hit a home run on Opening Day prompting a sportswriter to dub the new stadium 'The House that Ruth Built'. No truer words have ever been written in sports. Not only would there never had been a Yankee Stadium if Ruth did not exist but, the Yankees would not have become the legendary franchise it is today. In fact, baseball without Ruth, probably would not have become the popular game it is today in the United States and many other parts of the world. One could argue that Ruth actually saved the game itself as baseball might have not have survived the negative effects of a gambling scandal in which players were paid money to fix the outcome of the 1919 World Series.

Ruth's popularity off the field and larger-than-life exploits on the field made the public forget the dark shadow the scandal cast and enabled baseball to reach new heights of popularity.

Ruth's years with the Yankees were filled with world championships punctuated by legendary moments and gilded with incredible records. The many accomplishments of his baseball career were recognized by his induction, in the first-ever class, into the Baseball Hall of Fame in Cooperstown, New York in 1936.

Even though Babe became a worldwide celebrity, he never ceased to have time and energy for the ordinary person [5] especially children. During Babe's life he was dedicated to helping and providing comfort to the most vulnerable and forgotten individuals of society. He always had time for children- in particular, very ill children. Throughout his life Ruth would make countless visits to hospitals and orphanages around the world. On his visits to the hospitals, usually accompanied by his daughter, Dorothy, Babe would make sure that the first to be brought to see him would be the most ill because he knew that they would not live long enough to experience the joy of meeting him at the ballpark.

During winters in Sudbury, Massachusetts Babe would autograph multitudes of bats, balls, and gloves which his beloved daughter, Dorothy, would stockpile in the barn at Babe's 'Home Plate Farm'. Throughout the winter the stockpile would grow until the entire barn was filled with these autographed gifts that he would distribute to his many young fans during the upcoming baseball season. The huge stockpile would always be depleted by the time the baseball season was only a couple of months old. Babe would also invite orphanages over to his Sudbury farm. He would come out of the barn with wagons filled with baseball gifts for the little boys and dolls for the little girls.

When Babe would visit the children at various hospitals, he would be accompanied by his precious daughter, Dorothy, on these missions of mercy.

Dorothy would later say that when her 'Pop', as she called Babe, would enter a room the ill children would explode with happiness and delight. She described it as a magical experience where the children who couldn't sit up, sat up and those that couldn't run, ran [6].

To this day people visit Babe's grave at the Gate of Heaven Cemetery in Hawthorne, New York. They regularly leave tokens of their admiration for Babe along with requests that Babe aid them, from beyond the grave, in solving various issues and concerns in their own mortal lives.

NASOPHARYNGEAL CARCINOMA

Nasopharyngeal carcinoma (NPC) is a relatively rare tumor in many portions of the world such as the United States. However, it is the predominant form of cancer in certain areas such as the Arctic, Southeast Asia, southern China, North Africa, and the Middle East [7]. NPC arises from the epithelium of the nasopharynx which is the portion of the pharynx located above the soft palate.

A combination of radiation therapy and chemotherapy have been recommended as the preferred treatment modality for patients with advanced NPC [8-13]. For early-stage NPC radiotherapy alone is the current treatment approach [14].

NPC occurs more frequently in males and most commonly during an individual's sixth decade of life [15]. Risk factors for NPC include eating salted fish [16], viruses, genetic factors, and environmental factors [17]. It is important to note that, in whites in the United States, smoking and drinking have not been implicated as risk factors [18].

THE FINAL TWO YEARS

Ruth suffered through many misdiagnoses at various hospitals in New York City at the onset of his symptoms. In September of 1946 Ruth presented to the French Hospital with the left side of his face swollen and his left eye completely shut. He was diagnosed with either a toothache or sinusitis and his treatment consisted of penicillin and the extraction of three teeth. The misdiagnosis of sinusitis might have been due to the invasion of the tumor from the pterygoid muscles thus involving the maxillary sinus and orbits [19]. Obviously, the treatment Ruth received at the French Hospital gave him absolutely no relief from his suffering.

In November of 1946 his physicians, again at the French Hospital, diagnosed his condition as Horner Syndrome when a radiograph revealed a large mass at the base of his skull [19]. Babe was experiencing severe difficulty in chewing and dysphagia which may have been due to trismus as a result of the direct invasion of the medial or lateral pterygoid muscles and the involvement of certain cranial nerves which control swallowing movements and mastication [8].

Ruth was later misdiagnosed once again as having laryngeal carcinoma based on his supposed, but untrue, history of heavy alcohol and tobacco consumption. It is a fact that Babe used tobacco products but, he never smoked cigarettes. He was ahead of his time knowing that cigarettes would negatively affect an athlete's quality of play. Also, while Babe did drink alcohol from time to time, both the quantity and frequency of his alcohol use has been exaggerated by jealous detractors during his lifetime and poorly informed historians later who merely gave credence to erroneous statements.

By this time Ruth's internal carotid artery had been encircled by the tumor and might have invaded the cavernous sinus through the foramen lacerum thus causing opthalmoplegia [8].

Ruth underwent radiation therapy in November of 1946. In December of 1946, he underwent unsuccessful surgical resection of the tumor. This surgery left him unable to swallow thus requiring a feeding tube [19].

Babe would find some much sought-after relief from his suffering when he encountered Dr. Richard Lewisohn, a brilliant, forward-thinking physician. Dr. Richard Lewisohn was born on July 12, 1875 and received his medical education at the University of Freiburg [8]. Dr. Lewisohn made many contributions to medicine during his long career, primarily at New York's Mt. Sinai Hospital. His most well-known contribution is the introduction of the modern technique of blood transfusion [8]. In 1947, Dr. Lewisohn was experimenting with an anti-cancer drug, teropterin (pteroltriglutamic acid) [20]. However, to this point all his research was performed on mice. He was working with various teropterins, all of which were extracted from brewer's yeast. The particular preparation of the teropterin caused a wide variation in the effects seen on the mice [20]. Dr. Lewisohn offered Ruth to receive this experimental therapy. Dr. Lewisohn was very honest with Ruth about his chances for a recovery although no formal informed consent was signed. Dr. Lewisohn told Ruth that receiving this drug probably would not help him and, in fact, might even make his condition worse. Ruth responded bravely that he would still like to go through with the experimental treatment in order to provide the medical community with information that might help individuals in the future with the same ailment as his. Thus, Ruth became a subject in one of the first clinical trials of an anti-cancer drug [19]. Dr. Lewison's experimental course of teropterin injections led to a dramatic, albeit short- lived, improvement in Ruth. The improvement in Ruth's condition was featured in the lead story of September 11, 1947 in the Wall Street Journal which reported on Dr. Lewisohn's report of the case at a medical conference. The Wall Street Journal stated that researchers might be on the verge of a cure for cancer [21]. Ruth was able to say farewell to his fans at Yankee Stadium and attend other public functions as a direct result of Dr. Lewisohn's treatment.

Babe passed away on August 16, 1948. A wake was held at Yankee Stadium, 'The House the Ruth Built', and was attended by masses of people. The individuals were young and old, of all different nationalities, religions, and races. They certainly were not all baseball enthusiasts. Rather, they were people paying respect to a gentleman who dedicated his life to the well-being of others. Ruth did not have to constantly give of himself- of his time, his money, his efforts. He could have chosen to lead a very different life due to his almost superhuman ability on the baseball field. He made a choice most famous, wealthy athletes have not made. Ruth chose to give rather that to receive. Babe's funeral was at St. Patrick's Cathedral in New York City. As Babe's casket entered through the front doors of the Cathedral an eery silence blanketed the entire city. It was raining extremely hard during the funeral mass but the skies almost miraculously parted as the doors of St. Patrick's Cathedral opened and the casket was placed in a hearse for the journey to Gate of Heaven Cemetery in Hawthorne, New York. The approximately 30 mile route to the cemetery was lined with people six deep. One of these people was a blind man and his dog. Dorothy noticed them through the windows of the limousine. The blind man tapped the dog with a white cane as Babe's hearse drove by and the dog went to the ground and crossed his paws as if in prayer [22]. A graveside ceremony was held next to a stone which Dorothy picked out for her father. It was the biggest and most expensive stone in the entire cemetery. People still leave gifts and notes at this very stone to this day- paying tribute to the legacy of such a great man.

Babe fought a valiant two year battle against his own cancer. During this period he suffered tremendously and knew that his own death was near. Yet, the teachings which were instilled in him at St. Mary's remained with him to the end and Ruth selflessly continued his humanitarian mission. Cancer patients today directly benefit from the information researchers gathered from his case. Babe's wish came true- he is helping individuals with cancer today.

THE LEGACY

The story of Babe Ruth's life and legacy may have started on February 6, 1895 but, it certainly did not end on August 16, 1948 with his death. Babe, the Caliph of Clout, the Sultan of Swat, the Bambino- all nicknames for a mere mortal man. Ruth has been the subject of countless biographies, articles, cinematic representations and artistic renderings. Etymologically, Ruth's very name has become synonymous with 'superlative' and 'prodigiously accomplished'. The distinctive outline of Ruth swatting a mammoth blast or his facial likeness itself is ubiquitous over six decades after his death.

Ruth has become unquestionably a worldwide icon. However, even in stating this, one still does not adequately reflect the reverence with which his fans, or dare I even say, his disciples, view him. It must be stated that Ruth has transcended, in the public's eye, the limitations of mortal men. He has been placed by society amongst a very select few and continues to exert an influence upon and affect the living in a manner which is incongruous with that of a deceased individual. Ruth has almost achieved the age-old goal of man cheating death and thereby achieving immortality. Society has given him this gift of immortality. In return the conceptual notion of the benevolent figure aids society in coping with its own collective mortality.

Not only did Babe get his wish people today are directly benefitting from the cancer research performed on him but, his memory still influences individuals positively in the twenty-first century.

The adorable little girl who used to be in charge of her father's supply of gifts for the ill children grew into an extremely intelligent adult who carried on the charitable and inspiring works of her famous father long after his death. Before her own passing, Dorothy Ruth Pirone knew that a new generation would have to carry on the Ruthian legacy and was fortunate to have the perfect successor in her own daughter, Babe's granddaughter, Linda Ruth Tosetti. Today, Linda continues to give back to the people of the world while spreading the humanitarian message of her grandfather just as Babe would have wanted her to do.

REFERENCES

[1]   Babe Ruth. Available at: baberuthmuseum.org. Accessed on December 12, 2012.
[2]   Ettlin DM. Mamie Moberly, the Babe's sister, dies. The Baltimore Sun July 3, 1992.
[3]   Personal email communication on November 27, 2012 between William Maloney and Linda Ruth Tosetti.
[4]   'Ruth Bought by New York Americans for $125,000, Highest Price in Baseball Annals'. The New York Times. January 6, 1920.
[5]   Brooklyn Eagle Newspaper. March 2, 1922.
[6]   Personal email communication on August 5, 2012 between William Maloney and Linda Ruth Tosetti.
[7]   Chang ET, Adami HO. The enigmatic epidemiology of nasopharyngeal carcinoma. Cancer Epidemiol Biomarkers Prev 2006; 15(10): 1765-1777.
[8]   Maloney WJ, Weinberg MA. A comprehensive analysis of Baba Ruth's head and neck cancer. J Am Dent Assoc 2008 Jul; 139(7): 926-932.
[9]   Epstein JB, Emerton S, Lunn R, Le N, Wong FL. Pretreatment assessment and dental management of patients with nasopharyngeal carcinoma. Oral Oncol 1999; 35(1): 33-39.
[10]   Al-Sarraf M, LeBlanc M, Giri PG, *et al.* Chemoradiotherapy *versus* radiotherapy in patients with advanced nasopharyngeal cancer: phase III randomized Intergroup study 0099. J Clin Oncol 1998; 16(4): 1310-1317.
[11]   Rischin D, Corry J, Smith J, Stewart J, Hughes P, Peters L. Excellent disease control and survival in patients with advanced nasopharyngeal cancer treated with chemoradiation. J Clin Oncol 2002; 20(7): 1845-1852.

[12]   Dimery IW, Peters LJ, Goepfert H, *et al.* Effectiveness of combined induction chemotherapy and radiotherapy in advanced nasopharyngeal carcinoma. J Clin Oncol 1993; 11(10): 1919-1928.

[13]   Wee J, Tan EH, Tai BC, *et al.* Randomized trial of radiotherapy *versus* concurrent chemoradiotherapy followed by adjuvant chemotherapy in patients with American Joint Committee on Cancer/ International Union against cancer stage III and IV nasopharyngeal cancer of the endemic variety. J Clin Oncol 2005; 23(27): 6730-6738.

[14]   Caponigro F, Longo F, Ionna F, Perri F. Treatment approaches to nasopharyngeal carcinoma: a review. Anticancer Drugs. 2010 Jun, 21(5): 471-477.

[15]   Lee AW, Foo W, Mang O, *et al.* Changing epidemiology of nasopharyngeal carcinoma in Hong Kong over a 20-year period (1980-1999): an encouraging reduction in both incidence and mortality. Int J Cancer 2003; 103(5): 680-685.

[16]   Hareyama M, Sakata K, Shirato H, *et al.* A perspective, randomized trial comparing neoadjuvant chemotherapy with radiotherapy alone in patients with advanced nasopharyngeal carcinoma. Cancer 2002; 94(8): 2217-2223.

[17]   Chen CJ, Liang KY, Chang YS, *et al.* Multiple risk factors of nasopharyngeal carcinoma: Epstein-Barr virus, malarial infection, cigarette smoking and familial tendency. Anticancer Res 1990; 10(2B): 547-553.

[18]   Nam JM, McLaughlin JK, Blot WJ. Cigarette smoking, alcohol, and nasopharyngeal carcinoma: a case-control study among U.S. whites. J Natl Cancer Inst 1992; 84(8): 619-622.

[19]   Bikhazi NB, Kramer AM, Spiegel JH, Singer MI. "Babe" Ruth's illness and its impact on medical history. Laryngoscope 1999; 109(1): 1-3.

[20]   Ho JH. An epidemiologic and clinical study of nasopharyngeal carcinoma. Int J Radiat Oncol Biol Phys 1978; 4(3-4): 182-198.

[21]   Altman LK. The doctor's world: Ruth's other record—cancer pio- neer. N Y Times, Dec. 29, 1998: F1, F4. "http://query.nytimes.com/gst/ fullpage.html? res=9807E7DC143FF93A A15751C1A96E958260&sec=& spon=&pagewanted=2". Accessed May 15, 2008.

[22]   Personal email communication on August 21, 2012 between William Maloney and Linda Ruth Tosetti.

CHAPTER 4

Sigmund Freud's Medical Travails

Abstract: Oral cancer is the largest group of the subset of cancers which fall into the head and neck cancer category. It has multiple etiologies including tobacco and alcohol use. Alcohol seems to increase the odds for a malignancy to form in tobacco users. Sigmund Freud displayed a fervent addiction to tobacco. By Freud's own admission he was addicted to nicotine and was known to smoke twenty cigars per day. Freud documented in letters his desire to smoke cigars throughout his ordeal with oral cancer. A brief review of oral cancer will be discussed and details of Freud's struggle with the disease will be analyzed in this chapter.

Keywords: Alcohol, Anna Freud, biopsies, cancer surgery, cigars, electrocautery, graft, oral cancer, oral squamous cell carcinoma, prosthesis, resection, tobacco.

SIGMUND FREUD

Sigmund Freud was born in Frieberg, Moravia on May 6, 1856. Four years later his family moved to the city which Freud would become so deeply associated with for he rest of his life-Vienna. Upon graduating from the University of Vienna with a medical degree in 1881 Freud was employed as a physician at the Vienna General Hospital [1]. Early in his career, Freud had developed a deep interest in disorders which were considered to be of a nervous origin. He became very inspired by the work of a Viennese colleague, Josef Breuer, who had found that a hysterical patient would sometimes have their symptoms abated when allowed to talk in an uninhibited manner about the earliest occurrences of the symptoms.

Freud believed that neuroses originated from deeply traumatic experiences that had occurred in an individual's past. These occurrences had, in turn, been repressed and hidden from one's own consciousness. He felt that the way to treat such neuroses was to facilitate the patient in recalling the adverse experience and, in turn, analyzing this adverse experience both intellectually and emotionally. In so doing, Freud believed that the neurosis could be discharged. In 1895, Breuer and Freud published this theory in 'Studies in Hysteria'. Such groundbreaking work led to Freud becoming known as the 'father of psychoanalysis'.

ORAL CANCER

Head and neck cancers are the sixth most common malignancy worldwide and approximately half of these cases are squamous cell carcinomas (SCC) of the oral cavity [2, 3]. It is estimated that there are 300,000 new cases annually [4, 5]. The tongue is the most common site for this malignancy. The hard palate and the maxilla are much less common [5]. It has been documented that carcinoma of the hard palate is an uncommon malignancy that accounts for approximately five percent of all oral cancers [6]. The cause of this type of malignancy is varied and includes tobacco and alcohol use as well as a genetic predisposition. An additional and newly identified etiology is the human papilloma virus [7] which is also responsible for the vast majority of cervical cancers in women. Among men and women aged 14 to 69 years of age in the United States, the overall prevalence of oral HPV infection is 6.9%. The prevalence has been demonstrated to be higher among men than women [8].

Cigars, pipes and cigarettes have a dose-response relationship to oral, pharyngeal, and laryngeal cancer [2]. Oral squamous cell carcinoma has a varied clinical presentation including exophytic or endophytic growth and possibly being ulcerated with various color patterns such as leukoplakia or erythroplakia [9].

The treatment of patients with cancer does not cease with the elimination of the disease. Rehabilitation is an essential phase of cancer treatment and should be considered from the time of diagnosis [10]. Treatment of the patient with cancers of the maxilla and hard palate is complex and results in significant functional and esthetic sequelae [11-13]. These may include collapse of cheek and infraorbital soft tissues, loss of portions of the palate, and difficulty with articulation and orbital complications [11, 14]. These issues are often best controlled by employing a team approach utilizing multiple dental and medical specialties. Approximately 42,000 people in the United States alone will be newly diagnosed with oral cancer each year [7].

FREUD'S BATTLE WITH ORAL CANCER

"I began smoking at the age of 24, first cigarettes but soon exclusively cigars, and am still smoking now and very reluctant to restrict myself in this pleasure..." These are the words of Sigmund Freud, the father of psychoanalysis, who routinely smoked up to twenty cigars daily [3, 15].

During one period of abstinence, urged by his physician Dr. Fliess, Freud wrote "I have not smoked for seven weeks since the day of your injunction. At first I felt, as expected, outrageously bad. Cardiac symptoms accompanied by mild depression, as well as the horrible misery of abstinence. These wore off but left me completely incapable of working, a beaten man. After seven weeks I began smoking again ... Since the first few cigars, I was able to work and was the master of my mood; before that life was unbearable." [7]

At one point near the end of World War I cigars were difficult to obtain and Freud briefly ceased his smoking habit. During this period of tobacco abstinence, Freud recognized a painful swelling on his palate [15]. Numerous articles reported that Freud suspected a cancerous lesion but, nonetheless, he started smoking again and the lesion disappeared [3, 15, 16]. This fueled his reasoning that the lesion was psychogenic. He continued on with his career and personal life through the next six years without much concern for the recurring lesion on his palate. In February 1923 the lesion presented itself as an ulceration.

Procrastination continued to be Freud's trait concerning this malady. Two months passed until Freud visited two friends who were both physicians, Maxim Steiner and Felix Deutsch. Both of these practitioners suspected cancer but for reasons that can only be speculated upon, they deceived Freud and suggested leukoplakia and that the lesion required excision [16]. Max Schur, also a psychoanalyst, suggested that Deutsch could not face reality when he saw the aggressive lesion in Freud's mouth and was assailed by the horrifying conviction that this was not a leukoplakia but a malignant epithelioma [3]. Freud, suspecting cancer and upset over the deception "left the care of Deutsch" and sought an opinion from Marcus Hajek, Professor of Laryngology at Vienna University. Hajek (1861-1941) was renowned for his detailed knowledge of the para-nasal sinuses and originated the term 'Hajek's Triad' which describes the cause of nasal perforation as mucosal dryness, septal deviation, and infection. Dr. Hajek began a cascade of events when he recommended surgery to combat Freud's lesion which, by this time, Freud was referring to as "my dear neoplasm" [3, 16]. Hajek performed the surgery on an outpatient basis and poorly planned for the complications and sequelae that followed. Only partial excision of the lesion was accomplished and excessive hemorrhage during the procedure required Freud to be admitted to the hospital. The troubles continued as the hospital was full and Freud was placed into a small room which he was forced to share with a mentally disabled, deaf-mute dwarf. During the evening Freud experienced a second episode of hemorrhage and with Freud unable to speak the dwarf scouted the hospital until he found a nurse. He beckoned her back to the room where she successfully gained hemostasis. Anna, Freud's daughter, returned in the early morning to find her father sitting in a chair soaked with his own blood. She refused to leave his side. In the morning, Hajek performed his morning rounds but apparently paid little attention to Freud [3, 16]. The house pathologist confirmed the diagnosis of malignant epithelioma (squamous cell carcinoma) and Hajek recommended radiotherapy in addition to the unsuccessful surgery [16]. Freud briefly felt rejuvenated and described his passion for nicotine in a note to his friend, "I can again chew, work and smoke, and I shall try your optimistic slogan: many happy returns of the day and none of the new growth [16]. Unfortunately, his condition continued to deteriorate and, in 1923, Deutsch arranged an appointment for Freud to see Professor Hans Pichler [3, 16].

Hans Pichler studied dentistry under G.V. Black in Chicago at Northwestern University School of Dentistry. Upon his return to Vienna he embarked on a prominent career in oral surgery and was a noted author. He had a reputation as an aggressive, kind, and modest surgeon [16]. Pichler's approach to Freud's surgery was meticulous and well prepared. He proposed a two-stage surgery and practiced his technique on cadavers prior to the event [16, 17]. First, Pichler imposed a strict regimen of oral hygiene and treated any carious lesions and defective fillings. Gold inlays were placed in abutment teeth to support the planned maxillary obturator in order to obtain the best stability and comfort for the patient. The first part of the surgery took place in October of 1923 during which Pichler ligated the right external carotid artery to reduce bleeding. During the second stage he excised the right submandibular nodes.

This procedure was done with opium sedation and local anesthesia. In the second operation, during the month of October 1923, Pichler utilized electrocautery so any tumor cells in the line of the incision would be ablated. He reflected a facial flap and resected a large portion of the right maxilla. A portion of the coronoid process and part of the ramus of the mandible were also removed. A split thickness skin graft was obtained from Freud's upper arm. The maxillectomy cavity was then packed with iodoform gauze and the prosthesis fashioned by Pichler was inserted. After the operation, Pichler felt that his only mistake was that he hadn't removed enough of the medial pterygoid muscle. He was concerned that there would be a recurrence in that area. The pack was replaced after a week. Three weeks later, Pichler's concern became a reality when a small ulcer in the area of the right process was discovered. It was a recurrence confirmed by biopsy as being malignant [16]. Pichler fashioned an obturator prosthesis for Freud and performed a third resection. In 1924 Pichler documented seventy-four appointments for biopsies and prosthetics. Other dentists made additional prostheses. Freud was not fully satisfied. In total, Freud's lesion had recurrences and required more than 30 procedures until his death.

After sixteen years of battling this unrelenting disease process Sigmund Freud could continue no longer. The lesion had become so aggressive that it perforated his right cheek. The lesion became gangrenous [3]. Freud had a conversation with his trusted friend Max Schur when first diagnosed and asked him not to forsake him when the time came that the pain became intolerable [3, 15, 16]. The last words Freud spoke were to his friend and colleague Schur, "I thank you" and "tell Anna about this". All this was said without any trace of emotion or self-pity and with full consciousness of the reality of his situation [3]. His faithful friend dutifully injected two separate doses of morphine twelve hours apart and Freud fell into a peaceful sleep from which he would not awake.

REFERENCES

[1]   Tauber AI. Freud, the Reluctant Philosopher. Princeton University Press, 2010.
[2]   Schur M. Freud: Living and Dying. New York: International Universities Press, 1972.

[3]   Wolheim R. Sigmund Freud. Cambridge Univeristy Press, 1981.

[4]   Kademani D. Oral Cancer. Mayo Clinic Proc. 2007; 82: 878-887

[5]   Eskander A, Baback G, Gullane P, *et al*. Outcome Predictors in Squamous Cell Carcinoma of the Maxillary Alveolus and Hard Palate. The Laryngoscope. 2013; 00: 1-7

[6]   Krolls SO, Hoffman S. Squamous cell carcinoma of the oral soft tissues: a statistical analysis of 14,253 cases by age, sex, and race of patients. J Am Dent Assoc, 92 (1976), pp.571-574

[7]   Oral Cancer Foundation.org. Oral Cancer Facts. Available at: oralcancer.org/facts.indexhtml. Accessed on 5/2/13.

[8]   Gillison ML, Broutian T, Pickard RK, Tong ZY, Xiao W, Kahl L, Graubard BI, Chaturvedi AK. Prevalance of oral HPV infection in the U.S., 2009-2010, JAMA. 2012 Feb 15; 307(7): 693-703

[9]   Neville B, Damm D, Allen C, Bouquot J. Oral Maxillofacial Pathology. Third Edition. St. Louis MO: Elsevier/Saunders.

[10] Davenport JC. The Prosthetic Care of Sigmund Freud. Br Dent J 1992; 172: 205-207

[11] Fattah H, Zaghloul A, Pedemonte E, Escuin T. Pre-Prosthetic surgical alterations in maxillectomy to enhance the prosthetic prognosis as part of a rehabilitation of oral cancer patient. Med

[12] Adisma IK, Prosthesis serviceability for acquired jaw defects. Dent Clin North Am. 1990; 34: 265-84

[13] Wood RH, Carl W. Hollow silicone obturators for patients after total maxillectomy. J Prosthetic Dent. 1977; 38: 643-51

[14] Schusterman MA, Reece GP, Miller MJ. Osseous free flaps for orbit and midface reconstruction. Am J Surg. 1993; 116: 341-5

[15] Lazaridis N. Sigmund Freud's Oral Cancer. British Journal of Oral and Maxillofacial Surgery. 2003; 41: 78-83

[16] Davenport J. Sigmund Freud's Illness-The Ultimate Team Approach to Head and Neck Cancer? Facial Plastic Surgery. 1993; 9(2): 125-132

[17] Romm S, Luce E. Hans Pichler: Oral Surgeon to Sigmund Freud. Oral Surg Oral Med Oral Pathol. 1984 Jan; 57 (1): 31-32.

CHAPTER 5

Celiac Disease: The Cause of President John F. Kennedy's Life-Long Medical Travails

Abstract: John F. Kennedy was elected the first Roman Catholic president of the United States. His presidency lasted only approximately 1,000 days as he was assassinated in Dallas, Texas. During his lifetime, Kennedy suffered many ailments which baffled his physicians and led to numerous hospitalizations. Most prominent on the list of Kennedy's ailments were chronic back problems and gastrointestinal disorders. Kennedy was never diagnosed with celiac disease during his lifetime but such a diagnosis would explain his lifelong medical issues for which his physicians could not come up with a suitable diagnosis.

Celiac disease is an autoimmune disease in which there are many gastrointestinal manifestations such as diarrhea, weight loss, irritability, and abdominal pain.

Keywords: Abdominal pain, Addison's disease, adrenal crisis, autoimmune disease, barbituates, celiac disease, chronic back pain, codeine, colitis, demerol, diarrhea, gastrointestinal disorders, gluten, lomotril, osteoporosis, testosterone, weight loss.

JOHN F. KENNEDY

Between 1846 and 1849 approximately 100,000 Irish immigrants left their homeland and made their new home in Boston. These Irish immigrants had been forced to flee to Ireland due to the great potato famine. Boston provided a new home for these thousands of poor Irish families. The Irish immigrants faced many obstacles- discrimination, poverty, and disease- in their new, beloved nation to which they would be so loyal. In Mid-nineteenth century, Boston also provided something more than just a new home to these individuals. It provided a chance to the American dream- the opportunity to enjoy the fruits of their labor and, by means of strength of mind, body, and soul, to better their situation in life. For this alone, they were thankful.

In 1849, Patrick Kennedy and his wife, Bridget Murphy, disembarked from a passenger ship in Boston Harbor as they arrived in America from County Wexford, Ireland. They lived in a tiny apartment in East Boston. The couple eventually became the parents of four children. Nine years after arriving in America, Patrick died. Bridget became a 37 year-old widow with four children under the age of 8. Patrick had left her an estate valued at $75. The poverty-stricken yet, proud and strong widow became a servant. After some time she found work in a variety store. Eventually, Bridget bought the store [1].

On May 29, 1917, in nearby Brookline, Massachusetts, one of Patrick and Bridget's great-grandsons was born. The parents, Joseph and Rose Kennedy, would name their infant son John Fitzgerald Kennedy. This baby boy eventually became known to the entire world simply as JFK, 35th president of the United States. He became a war hero in 1943 when his small PT boat was rammed and sunk by a Japanese destroyer and later, as president, was loved and admired by millions worldwide and lead the nation through the crucial days of the Cuban Missile Crisis. He inspired America to literally reach for the stars by championing the space program with his words, "We choose to go to the moon in this decade, and do the other things, not because they are easy, but because they are hard ..."

JFK's life would end in Dallas, Texas on November 22, 1963- one of the darkest days in American history. In the years since his death, JFK has become an iconic figure still inspiring individuals around the globe today.

CELIAC DISEASE

Celiac disease (CD) is a chronic systemic autoimmune disease which occurs in genetically susceptible individuals. It was first recognized in 1887 [2]. Its prevalence is between 1% and 2% of the population in some nations [3]. There are a number of gastrointestinal manifestations of this disorder such as diarrhea, weight loss, abdominal pain, and irritability [4]. Some individuals with CD do not have diarrhea or weight loss. These individuals have iron deficiencies or alterations in blood chemistry [3].

Celiac disease damages the villi of the small intestine. The villi, in health, act to absorb vitamins, minerals, and various other nutrients. In CD the villi are damaged resulting in the malabsorption of nutrients which are required for health and growth [5]. CD is difficult to diagnose because it resembles several other conditions that can cause malabsorption.

The immune system of an individual with CD may be identifying gluten as a foreign substance and producing elevated levels of antibodies to rid the body of it [6]. Most individuals with CD have celiac disease-associated antibodies and specific pairs of allelic variants in two HLA genes, HLA-DQA1 and HLA-DQB1 [7].

There have been various case reports in the medical literature demonstrating a link between CD and Addison's disease. O'Leary *et al.* [6] have shown, in a series of patients with Addison's disease, there to be a higher co-morbidity with CD than in any previously studied endocrine condition. It is strongly suggested that individuals with Addison's disease be tested for CD.

The diagnosis of CD is achieved by two specific and sequential criteria [3]. Firstly, prior to treatment there needs to be shown typical biopsy changes in the proximal small intestine. Secondly, there needs to be a definitive clinical and/or pathological response to a particular diet. Foods which may contain gluten include breads, biscuits, cakes, pastries, pizza, pasta, sausage meats, certain soups, certain gravies, certain breakfast cereals and certain sauces [7]. Gluten-free foods include unprocessed fruit, vegetables, milk, eggs, rice, fish, and meat [7].

In the future, new forms of treatment for CD may include the use of substrates which regulate intestinal permeability to prevent gluten entry across the epithelium, different forms of immunotherapy, the development of gluten-free grains by genetic modification, and the use of gluten-degrading enzymes [8].

Population-based screening studies have demonstrated a higher prevalence of CD in Ireland than elsewhere in the world [9]. This prevalence rate is slightly less than 1% of the population. Mylotte *et al.* [10] demonstrated a high prevalence of CD in workers in Galway in 1973. The genetic stock of the Irish people is thought to have been established approximately 5,000 years ago [9, 11] before the arrival of the Celts. It is thought that the ethnic and genetic mix is homogenous and distinct relative to much of mainland Europe [9]. From prehistoric times to the great potato famine of the nineteenth century, oats were the only cereal and source of gluten consumed for most of the population of Ireland [9]. Presently, the Irish diet differs little from the rest of western civilization. Cronin [9, 11] states that until only very recently the Irish diet has almost been gluten-free and postulates that there is a suggestion that the possession of CD genes in areas of low gluten consumption must confer a survival advantage and thus explains the high prevalence of CD in the modern day Irish who have only recently been exposed to such a wide variety of food with a high gluten content.

KENNEDY'S LIFELONG MEDICAL ORDEALS

For over half a century the extensive medical history of President John F. Kennedy has remained hidden from the public. Recently, historians have been granted limited access to his medical records from the John F. Kennedy Presidential Library in Boston, Massachusetts. These records have shed new light on the health of the President while raising new questions.

Kennedy's presidency was characterized by the vibrancy, vigor and well-being of the youthful President and his family. Images of the young President enjoying outdoor physical activities along the shore of his family's home in Cape Cod filled the American imagination with the hope of a bright new future for the nation. Legendary stories abounded with his exploits on the football field and his heroism at war. Were these images merely casual glimpses of an energetic and vibrant American president in the prime of his life enjoying his youthful and appealing family or was it more accurately a carefully choreographed view of a man with great political aspirations and a will of iron which enabled him to hide his intense chronic physical pain from the unsuspecting public's eye?

Among the litany of Kennedy's physical ailments were constant back pain and severe bouts of diarrhea which would leave him hospitalized for weeks at a time. These symptoms, along with his Irish heritage and small physical stature as a youth, point towards an undiagnosed case of Celiac disease (CD) (Table **3**). CD is an autoimmune digestive disease which is characterized by the malabsorption of nutrients. Also, Kennedy's well- documented Addison's disease lends even more credence to the theory that many of his debilitating physical ailments were due to an undiagnosed case of CD. Individuals with Addison's disease have a much higher incidence of CD than the rest of the population. Also, CD is much more prevalent in individuals of Irish ancestry. Kennedy's ancestors, living in Ireland, probably would not have been aware that they possessed the gene predisposing them to CD as they were exposed to a diet that was primarily gluten-free. It is gluten food products that bring on the symptoms of CD and the only treatment of the disease presently is a gluten-free diet.

Table 3. Signs and Symptoms of Celiac Disease

-anemia
-loss of bone density
-abdominal bloating
-weight loss
-joint pain
-damage to dental enamel
-acid reflux
-fatigue
-vomiting
-irritability

President Kennedy spent many days in the hospital searching for the cause of and some relief from his gastrointestinal woes. No relief was found and no relief is to be expected in an individual suffering from CD until a gluten-free diet is instituted. Eventually, CD can lead to back pain due to the collapse of the lumbar vertebrae [12]. President Kennedy's chronic back problems have been known to the American public since his presidency. The extent and cause of this pain have remained in the shadows throughout the years. Kennedy's advisors sought to explain his back ailments with stories of heroism on the football field and aboard PT 109 in the Pacific. In recent years, the public has become more aware of the Addison's disease of President Kennedy. It has not been until recently that historians and the public have become aware of the voluminous nature of Kennedy's medical records. Throughout his life, Kennedy's hospitalizations were numerous and often. His hospitalizations ranged from being diagnostic in nature to life-threatening. Above all, it was imperative to Kennedy and his advisors that the grave and debilitating nature of his illnesses remain an absolute secret from the American public so as not to raise questions as to whether he was medically able to withstand the rigors and pressures that go with being the occupant of the Oval Office.

A physician on the White House staff, Admiral George Burkley, was so intent on giving the impression that Kennedy was in excellent health that he avoided having "a medical man in the near proximity to him" in public [13].

John Kennedy's medical maladies started in the 1920's when he was a young child. He suffered from German measles, mumps, whooping cough, chicken pox, bronchitis, and ear infections [13]. In April of 1931, Kennedy collapsed from abdominal pains and was misdiagnosed with appendicitis at a hospital in Danbury, Connecticut. Surgery was performed and, obviously, no relief was found. He was also, at this time, not successful in gaining much needed weight to his almost gaunt frame. In the winter of 1934 he was rushed in an ambulance to New Haven Hospital for observation due to his weight loss and hives. Now doctors suspected leukemia [13].

By 1937, Kennedy started taking corticosteroids to relieve his colitis. Long-term effects of their use include osteoporosis, skin that turns the yellow-gold of a permanent suntan, hair that stays thick and dark, and an increased sex drive- all of which describe the physical traits of John Kennedy [14].

Kennedy visited England in September of 1947 as a congressman from Massachusetts. During this visit, he collapsed and the admitting physician, Sir Daniel Davis, diagnosed adrenal crisis. Davis told a friend of Kennedy, Pamela Churchill, "That young American friend of yours, he hasn't got a year to live" [10, 15]. This episode was explained to the public by saying that it was a severe recurrence of the malaria he had contracted in the Pacific during World War II [16]. Kennedy survived this episode and was hospitalized nine times between 1955 and 1957 for back and intestinal ailments [17]. He denied any rumors of his Addison's disease to the public [18]. "I have never had the matter to which you referred, Addison's disease." [19].

During his presidency, Kennedy was taking antispasmodics for his colitis; antibiotics for a urinary tract infection; hydrocortisone, testosterone, and salt tablets for his adrenal insufficiency and to boost his energy; lomotil for diarrhea; stelazine, meprobamate, and librium for anxiety; codeine, demerol, and methadone for pain; barbituates for sleep; a thyroid hormone; ritalin- a stimulant; gamma globulin to combat infections; and 7 to 8 daily injections of procaine at one time for his back pain [19].

From analyzing Kennedy's complete medical history, a presumptive diagnosis of CD can be made by analyzing the following six factors: 1) Irish heritage, 2) the development of Addison's disease, 3) diagnosis of irritable bowel syndrome, 4) diagnosis of migraine, 5) presence of gastrointestinal complaints since childhood, and 6) presence of severe osteoporosis [3]. Frozen blood samples or certain preserved biopsy materials could confirm the diagnosis of CD today [3].

A diagnosis of CD is the missing link in understanding Kennedy's life-long battle against his physical ailments. It puts to rest the myth and imagery of his back problems being a mere side effect of 'playing football' or 'a war injury'.

A diagnosis of CD should not diminish President Kennedy's accomplishments. It might even make his star shine brighter now that the American public knows how rationally and adeptly he handled the many crucial issues he faced during his presidency while enduring his own intense physical pain. Only now, through his pain, can we truly understand the President as a real and visceral man.

REFERENCES

[1]   Leamer L. The Kennedy Men: 1901-1963. New York: William Morrow, 2001.
[2]   Green PHR. Was JFK the victim of an undiagnosed disease common to the Irish? 2010. Available at: http://hnn.us/articles/1125.html.
[3]   Freeman HJ. Adult celiac disease and its malignant complications. Gut and Liver December 2009; 3(4): 237-246.
[4]   Snyder CL, Young DO, Green PHR, Taylor AK. Celiac disease. 2010. Available at: http://www.ncbi.nih.gov/bookshelf/br.fcgi?book=gene∂=celiac.
[5]   Mayo Clinic. 2010. Available at: http://www.mayoclinic.com/health/celiac-disease/ds00319/dsection=symptomsrash.
[6]   O'Leary C, Walsh CH, Wieneke P, *et al*. Coeliac disease and autoimmune Addison's disease: a clinical pitfall. QJM 2002 Feb; 95(2): 79-82.
[7]   Coeliac Society of Ireland. 2010. Available at: http://www.coeliac.ie/ coeliacdisease.htm.
[8]   Setty M, Hormaza L, Guandalini S. Celiac disease: risk assessment, diagnosis, and monitoring. Mol Diagn Ther 2008; 12(5): 289-298.

[9]   Cronin CC, Fergus S. Why is celiac disease so common in Ireland? Pers Biol Med Summer 2001; 44(3): 342-352.

[10]   Mylotte M, *et al*. Incidence of coeliac disease in the west of Ireland. BMJ 1973; 1: 703-705.

[11]   de Paor L. The people of Ireland. In The people of Ireland, edited by P. Loughrey. 185-189. Belfast: Appletree, 1988.

[12]   Celiac Sprue Association. 2010. Available at: http://www.csacelics.org/celiac- symptoms.php

[13]   Dallek R. The medical ordeals of JFK 2010. Available at: http:// www.theatlantic.com/magazine/print/2002/12/the-medical-ordeals-of-jfk/5572/.

[14]   Lacayo R. How sick was J.F.K.? 2010. Available at: http://www.time.com/time/printout/0,8816,1003773,00.html.

[15]   Blair J, Blair C. The Search for JFK. New York: Berkley; 1976: 561.

[16]   Mandel LR. Endocrine and autoimmune aspects of the health history of John F. Kennedy. Annals of Internal Medicine 1 September 2009; 151(5): 350-354.

[17]   Altman LK, Purdum TS. In J.F.K. file, hidden illness, pain and pills 2010. Available at: http://www.nytimes.com/2002/11/17/politics/17JFK.html?pagewanted=1&pagewanted=print.

[18]   Loughlin KR. John F. Kennedy and his adrenal disease. Urology 2002; 59: 165-169.

[19]   New York Times, November 10, 1960, p 37.

CHAPTER 6

Porphyria: The Cause of the Madness of King George

Abstract: King George III was the reigning monarch of Great Britain who had his troops vanquished by the colonial forces during the American War for Independence. At age 50, George III began experiencing various symptoms including insomnia, stupor, restlessness, and headaches. His systems disappeared and he mysteriously recovered. Symptoms returned over a decade later and eventually led to King George III losing the royal throne. Modern research shows that the cause of King George III's illness was porphyria. Porphyrias are a group of rare diseases. This group of diseases is characterized by an enzyme deficiency in the heme biosynthesis pathway.

Keywords: Constipation, convulsions, dark red urine, delirium, fever, heme, insanity, insomnia, low blood pressure, parliament, porphyria, stupor, tachycardia, visual problems, weak limbs.

KING GEORGE III

On June 4, 1738 George III was born to Frederick, Prince of Wales, and Princess Augusta of Saxe-Gotha. He was their first born child. His grandfather was King George II, monarch of the United Kingdom [1].

In 1761, George and Charlotte of Mecklenburg-Strelitz were married. The marriage produced 15 children. During George's reign he became vilified and saw the crown beset by much financial difficulties. Many of his problems were caused by his appointment of the Earl of Bute as his first chief minister.

The Earl of Bute isolated the King from his senior politicians. The Earl eventually resigned in 1763. However, the King's problems certainly did not end there. Rather, George III's problems were actually just beginning.

The Seven Years' War did much to continue to deplete the British financial resources.

In order to rectify the British debt problem, Parliament enacted new taxes. The American colonists resented the additional taxes and the lack of liberties which other British subjects enjoyed. George III never thought that this disharmonious situation would come to war [2]. The American colonists fought for their independence and would eventually win the long and bloody war. George III hoped for a British victory until the spectacular British defeat at Yorktown in October 1781. The House of Commons would then vote to suspend military operations in North America.

Eventually George III accepted destiny's desire when he stated to John Adams, the first ambassador of a sovereign United States of America, that he desired to "meet the friendship of the United States as an independent power" [3].

On January 9, 1820 King George III died. He was buried in St. George's Chapel, Windsor Castle [4].

PORPHYRIA

Porphyrias refer to a group of rare disorders which arise from a disruption in the body's production of heme. They consist of eight genetically distinct metabolic disorders [5]. There are certain enzymes in the body which convert porphyrins to heme. A mutation in one of the genes which is involved in heme production can result in an enzyme deficiency which, in turn, leads to the accumulation of porphyrins in the body [6]. Presently there are DNA-based diagnoses for all the porphyrias [5]. Porphyrias are classified as being either hepatic or erythropoietic porphyrias. The hepatic porphyrias include acute intermittent porphyria, hereditary coproporphyria, variegate porphyria, aminolevulnic acid dehydratase deficiency porphyria and porphyria cutanea tarda while the erythropoietic porphyrias include uroporphyria and protopoporphyria [7].

The symptoms of the porphyrias include light sensitivity, abdominal pain, neurological and muscular disturbances, muscle pain, muscle weakness or paralysis, numbness or tingling, pain in the arms or legs, pain in the back, personality changes, low blood pressure, severe electrolyte imbalances, and shock [8].

There are many causes of porphyria such as drugs, infections, estrogen, and alcohol [8]. Most forms of porphyria are inherited. They can either exhibit an autosomal dominant pattern or an autosomal recessive pattern [6].

Tests used in the diagnosis of porphyrias usually measure substances which accumulate in large quantities in the body. These porphyrin precursors and porphyrins can be measured in feces, urine, red blood cells, and blood plasma [9]. Other diagnostic tests which may aid in the diagnosis are blood gases, comprehensive metabolic panel, ultrasound of the abdomen and urinalysis [8].

Treatments of porphyrias include intravenously administered hematin, pain medication, propanolol to control the heartbeat, sedatives, beta-caroten supplements, fluids and glucose and, in the case of life-threatening acute attacks, liver transplantation [8]. Attacks and symptoms of porphyrias are transient. They appear and disappear over the course of an individual's life. Avoidance of certain triggers can prolong the interval between attacks.

THE EFFECT OF PORPHYRIA ON KING GEORGE III

For centuries, the 'madness' of King George III has intrigued politicians, historians, biographers, and medical experts. His illness had dramatic effects on his nation. This has, of course led to much speculation as to what was at the root of the King's malady. Most modern scientific evidence and analyses point towards a case of porphyria.

King George III was struck down five times by episodes of madness with two recurrences being particularly dramatic and chaotic for the British government [10, 11]. King George III's first symptoms appeared when he was 50 years-old. Initially, he experienced constipation, and abdominal pain which was followed by fever, tachycardia, weak limbs, dark red urine, and hoarseness, These symptoms were soon followed by headaches, insomnia, delirium, convulsions, stupor, and visual problems. He would rip off his wig and run naked through the royal courts. Obviously, Parliament did not look favorably on their monarch's behavior and was debating his ability to rule when he mysteriously and suddenly recovered [12].

The King would relapse 13 years later and suffer other relapses in subsequent years. He was left in a permanent stupor by an attack of his ailment in 1811. At this point he was dethroned by the Prince of Wales [12].

In December 1810, Dr. Robert Darling Willis was asked to summarize the King's health problems by a parliamentary committee to which he would state, "I would consider the King's derangement more nearly allied to delirium ... In delirium, the mind is actively employed upon past impressions ... which rapidly pass in succession ... There is also a considerable disturbance in the general constitution; great restlessness, great want of sleep, and total unconsciousness of surrounding objects. In insanity, there may be little or no disturbance, apparently, in the general constitution; the mind is occupied upon some fixed assumed idea ... and the individual is acting, always, upon that false impression ... also, the mind is awake to objects which are present. Taking insanity, therefore, and delirium, as two points, I would place derangement of mind somewhere between them. His Majesty's illness, uniformly, partakes more of the delirium than of insanity [12]."

It has been theorized [13] that the particular form of porphyria which afflicted King George III is acute intermittent porphyria. Acute intermittent porphyria is transmitted *via* Mendellian dominant inheritance thus causing the expectancy of seeing other family members affected. This was true in the case of George III's youngest sister, Caroline Matilda, Queen of Denmark and Norway. She started experiencing general malaise which was followed rapidly by the paralysis of her arms and legs along with tachycardia. She started to exhibit symptoms at the same time as her brother [10, 13, 14].

Recently, in a London museum, a scrap of paper was found. This piece of paper had been folded to form a crude envelope. Written on the paper were the words: "Hair of His Late Majesty, King George 3rd." The hair was taken to Harwell International Business Centre for Science & Technology in Didcot, Oxfordshire for analysis. The results were astounding. The hair was laden with arsenic at a level 300 times higher than the toxic level. Arsenic is known to trigger porphyria [15].

The King had ingested arsenic over the first part of his life as arsenic is found in skin cream and wig powder. When symptoms of George III's ailment started to occur he was given liberal doses of a medicine referred to as James' powders. James' powders is made of antimony. Ironically, the medication used to control the 'madness' brought on by exposure to arsenic contained massive amounts of arsenic thus sealing the King's fate.

REFERENCES

[1]   The British Monarchy. George III (r. 1760-1820). Accessed on 8/4/12. Available at: http://www.royal.gov.uk/historyofthemonarchy/kingsandqueensoftheunitedkingdom/thehanoverians/georgeiii.aspx.
[2]   BBC. George III (1738-1820). Accessed on September 15, 2013. Available at: http://www.bbc.co.uk/history/historic_figures_iii_king.shtml/
[3]   The Examiner. The Colonists: King George III and the American Revolution Part One. Accessed on September 4, 2013. Available at: http://www.examiner.com/article/ the-colonists-king-george-iii-and-the-american-revolution-part-one.
[4]   Baer M. George III (1738-1820). Accessed on September 16, 2013. Available at: http://www.encyclopediavirginia.org/George_III_1738-1820#start_entry.
[5]   Balwani M, Desnick RJ. The Porphyrias: advances in diagnosis and treatment. Blood. 2012 Jul 12. [Epub ahead of print].
[6]   Mayo Clinic. Porphyria. Accessed on July 23, 2013. Available at: www.mayoclinic.com/health/porphria/DS00955.
[7]   Song HW, Shin YH, Ko JS, Gwak MS, Kim GS. A Case report of anesthesia management in the liver transplantation recipient with porphyria. Korean J Anesthesiol 2012 January 62(1): 83-86.
[8]   U.S. National Library of Medicine. Acute intermittent porphyria; Hereditary coproporphyria; congenital erythropoietic porphyria; erythropoietic protoporphyria. A.D.A.M. Medical Encyclopedia. Atlanta (GA): A.D.A.M.; 2011.
[9]   American Porphyria Foundation. About Porphyria. Accessed on June 4, 2012. Available at: www.porphyriafoundation.com/about-porphyria.
[10]   Macalpine I and Hunter R. The "Insanity" of King George III: a Classic Case of Porphria. Brit Med J 1966; 1: 65-71.
[11]   Ray I. "Insanity of King George III." Amer J Insan, 12, 1. Reprinted at the Asylum, Utica, 1855; in Forbes Winslow's J. psychol. Med. ment. Path., 10, 95. Translated by H. Laehr in Allg. Z. Psychiat, 1861, 18, 407. Republished with additions in Contributions to Mental Pathology. Little, Brown, Boston, 1873.
[12]   Report from the Committee Appointed to Examine the Physicians who have attended His Majesty, during His Illness, touching the State of His Majesty's Health. House of Commons, December 1788.
        -House of Lords, December 1788
        -House of Commons, January 1789
        -House of Commons, November 1810

-House of Commons, December 1810

-House of Lords, December 1810

-House of Commons, January 1812

[13]   Wraxall, Sir N.W. (1799). Memoirs of the Court of Berlin, Dresden, Warsaw, and Vienna. Cadell and Davies, London.

[14]   Wraxall, Sir C. F. L. (1864). Life and Times of Her Majesty Queen Caroline Matilda. Allen, London.

[15]   BBC News. King GeorgeIII: Mad or Misunderstood? Accessed on April 10, 2012. Available at: news.bbc.co.uk/2/hi/3889903.stm.

CHAPTER 7

President William Taft and Sleep Apnea

Abstract: William Taft was the 27th president of the United States. Much of the story of his medical travails centers upon one thing-his weight. Taft moved up the political ladder relatively quickly but, was never happy in politics. He was pushed by his father and his wife to reach great heights in politics. He would have rather simply practiced law. Taft's weight caused him to develop sleep apnea. After his term as president ended, he almost immediately lost approximately 70 pounds permanently. His sleep apnea disappeared as he lost the weight.

Keywords: Blood pressure, depression, history, macroglossia, neck circumference, obesity, sleep apnea, small mandible size, snoring, somnolence.

PRESIDENT WILLIAM TAFT

William Howard Taft was born on September 15, 1857 in Cincinnati, Ohio. He was born into a very respected family. His father, Alphonso Taft, has great expectations for the newborn child and was very demanding on him throughout his childhood in an effort to see that he became a success in life. Alphonso Taft was a prominent Cincinnati Republican and a distinguished attorney. He had served as secretary of war and then, subsequently as attorney general under President Ulysses S. Grant. Under President Chester Arthur he served as the United States Ambassador to Austria-Hungary and Russia [1].

William Howard Taft eventually attended and graduated from Yale University. Upon graduation he returned to Cincinnati to study and practice law [2]. Although Taft rose quickly in politics due to various Republican judiciary appointments he continued to favor law to politics. He was appointed a Federal Circuit judge at the age of 34 and aspired to become a member of the United States Supreme Court. However, his wife, Helen Herron Taft, held ever loftier aspirations for him.

Taft was eventually appointed chief civil administrator of the Phillipines by President William McKinley and as secretary of war by President Theodore

Roosevelt. In 1907 President Roosevelt decided that Taft should be his successor as President of the United States [2]. Taft was not very popular during his presidency because of his narrow interpretation of presidential powers [3] and the lack of ideological passion which contrasted poorly with the dynamic imperialistic style of Theodore Roosevelt.

After leaving the White House, Taft was free to purse his true love-law. he served as Professor of Law at Yale University and was later appointed by President Harding as Chief Justice of the United States Supreme Court. He held this position until his death in 1930.

Upon being appointed as Chief Justice, Taft wrote "I don't remember that I ever was President" [6].

SLEEP APNEA

Obstructive sleep apnea syndrome is a clinical medical condition which is characterized by irregular breathing at night combined with excessive daytime sleepiness [4]. Disorders which predispose to the stenosis of the upper airways and to the reduction of their stability cause an increased risk of obstructive sleep apnea [4, 5]. The most cited risk factor is obesity. Other risk indicators include a neck circumference higher than 43 cm, macroglossia, small mandible size, depression, male gender, reduction of nasal patency, obstruction of the upper airway due to any cause, increased tonsillar size, sedative drugs, increasing age, smoking, and alcohol use [4, 7].

The best way to diagnose obstructive sleep apnea is by having the patient complete an overnight sleep study in a laboratory [8]. The study includes electroencephalography, electrooculography, sleep positions, oxygen saturations, electrocardiography, electromyography, and respiratory activity [9].

Today, the care of sleep apnea patients entails a team approach consisting of many varied healthcare professionals. Dentistry plays a significant role in co-managing patients with simple snoring and mild to moderate obstructive sleep apnea. Dentists aid in the recognition of a sleep-related disorder, the referral process, and the actual management of the sleep disorder [10].

TAFT'S MEDICAL TRAVAILS

During President William Howard Taft's term in the White House (1909-1913) he suffered from obstructive sleep apnea evidenced by snoring, systemic hypertension, excessive daytime somnolence and perhaps cognitive and psychosocial impairment [11].

Taft weighed between 300 and 332 pounds [12, 13]. During his presidency he had a very difficult time staying awake even during the most serious of situations. He was observed to have fallen asleep during meetings with the Speaker of the House, the Chief Justice of the Supreme Court, and the wife of the French ambassador [14]. This daytime somnolence prompted Senator James Watson to write "Most of the time [Taft] simply did not and could not function in alert fashion ... Often when I was talking to him after a meal his head would fall over on his breast and he would go sound asleep for ten or fifteen minutes. He would awaken and resume the conversation, only to repeat the performance in the course of half an hour or so." [15]

By 1910 Taft had weighed in at 330 pounds [16]. An aide to the President stated that "he pants for breath at every step" [16].

He was examined by Dr. James Marsh Jackson of Boston, Massachusetts. The President wrote a letter, in 1914, describing his physical examination by Dr. Jackson. It was typed and read "I met Dr. Jackson, of Boston, when I was up there last week. He had examined me in the summer of 1910 or 1911, and took my blood pressure and had my urine examined and all the things you Doctors do to a man. I asked him to send you a record that he had made, for your record. You see I am determined to give you all available data. I send this that you may understand his writing you." Taft concluded, in his own handwriting, "He said my blood pressure was 210- whew! [17]".

Taft tolerated the jokes about his weight very well. A friend of his, Anson Phelps Stokes, who was Secretary of Yale University asked the President, in 1912, that he occupy a Chair of Law at Yale after his White House days. Taft responded that "a chair would not be adequate, but that if we could provide a Sofa of Law, it might be all right [18]."

Mrs. Taft and the presidential physicians were concerned about Taft's growing health issues related to his weight and did everything possible to curtail the President's eating habits.

However, when Taft went on overnight trips he was in command of his culinary choices. On one train trip through Pennsylvania, Taft was disturbed that there was no dining car on the train.

He roared "I am President of the United States and I want a diner attached to this train at Harrisburg. I want it well stocked with food, including filet mignon. You see that we get a diner. What's the use of being President if you can't have a train with a diner on it?" [18]

Taft never enjoyed politics. This was clearly evident in his years in the White House. His true love was law. Within 12 months of leaving the White House Taft lost almost 70 pounds permanently and his sleep apnea disappeared [11]. He lived an active and fairly healthy life for 17 years after his presidency, serving in the position he so loved and cherished- Chief Justice of the United States- until the day he died.

REFERENCES

[1]   Miller Center. American President: A Reference Resource. Accessed on 7/26/13. Available at: http://millercenter.org/president/taft/essays/biography/ AmericanPresident: AReferenceResource.
[2]   The White House. William Howard Taft. Accessed on 7/12/13. Available at: http://m.whitehouse.gov/about/presidents/williamhowardtaft.
[3]   PBS. William Howard Taft. accessed on March 26, 2013. Available at: http://millercenter.org/president/taft/essays/biography/ AmericanPresident: AReferenceResorce.
[4]   Conti AA, Conti A, and Gensini GF. Fat snorers and sleepy-heads: were many distinguished characters of the past affected by the obstructive sleep apnea syndrome? Medical Hypotheses 2006; 67(4): 975-979.
[5]   Clinical evidence, vol. 15. BMJ Publishing Group: 2006.
[6]   Jung R, and Kuhlo W. Neurophysiological studies of abnormal sleep and the Pickwickian syndrome. Prog Brain Res 1965; 18: 140-1559.
[7]   Andrews JG, and Oei TPS. The roles of depression and anxiety in the understanding and treatment of obstructive sleep apnea syndrome. Clin Psychol Rev 2004; 24: 1031-1049.

[8]   Magliocca KR, and Helman JI. Diagnosis, medical management and dental implications. Obstructive sleep apnea. J Am Dent Assoc 2005; 136(8): 1121-1129.

[9]   Polkey MJ, Morrell MJ, and Simonds AK. Apnea and history. Chest 2004; 125: 1587.

[10]   Padma A, Ramakrishnan N, Narayanan V. Management of obstructive sleep apnea: a dental perspective. Indian J Dent Res 2007; 18: 201-209.

[11]   Sotos JG. Taft and Pickwick: sleep apnea in the White House. Chest 2003; 124(3): 1133-1142.

[12]   Coletta PE. The Presidency of William Howard Taft. 1973, 1 University of Kansas Press. Lawrence, KS: 53.

[13]   Taft Reaches City. Washington Post. February 28, 1909, 1.

[14]   Butt AW. Taft and Roosevelt: the intimate letters of Archie Butt, military aide 1930; Doubleday; Doran. Garden City, NY.

[15]   Watson JE. I knew them: memoirs of James E Watson 1936, 134-135 Bobbs- Merrill. Indianapolis, IN.

[16]   Sotos JG. President Taft's Blood Pressure. Mayo Clinic Proc 2006; 81(11): 1507-1508.`

[17]   William Howard Taft papers, Library of Congress. Letter from Taft to Dr. George Blumer. January 18, 1914.

[18]   New York Magazine. Accessed on June 1, 2013. Available at: http://nymag.com/ daily/intelligencer/2013/02/chris-christie-william-howard-taft-weight-fat.hml.

CHAPTER 8

Pott's Disease: The Childhood Disease of Timothy Cratchit

Abstract: Charles Dickens is known throughout the world as perhaps the greatest novelist of all time. Dickens was highly interested in many social causes during his lifetime. One such cause was access to quality medical care for children. 20th century renovations at a London church revealed a tomb containing the body of an individual who served as the inspiration for his most beloved character, Timothy Cratchit or, more famously, 'Tiny Tim.'

Cratchit's skeletal remains were not that of a young boy but, rather, that of an adult. By virtue of this information, Dickens' 'A Christmas Carol' must be viewed as a social commentary. The hidden message of 'A Christmas Carol' is that children have the ability to overcome devastating physical ailments and handicaps if the proper medical care is provided.

Keywords: A Christmas Carol, Cratchit, grave, lumbar vertebrae, Pott's Disease, Royal Historic Society, Scrooge, Sir Percivall Pott, spine, thoracic vertebrae, tuberculosis.

TINY TIM

In 1963 workers paved over graves and grave markers at St. Andrew's Church in London. These graves and markers had already been long forgotten by modern society having had debris strewn about them for many years. In 1997, construction workers uncovered these graves while conducting excavations to strengthen the buttresses and roof supports of the church [1]. Uncovering long-forgotten graves in this particular section of London is no unique or noteworthy occurrence. Construction crews regularly uncover lost graves. However, the Royal Historic Society was summoned to assess the graves potential archeological value. They removed some rather large stones to reveal a grave with the skeletal remains of a male individual who had passed away in 1884.

The skeleton was still wearing a metal and leather frame on his legs and lower back as this individual had worn during his lifetime. Why would this individual be buried with this medical device that this man had to wear during his life? Was it a clue to a deeper connection between the man whose remains lay in this grave and something more meaningful than merely an uncomfortable but much needed medical device which had lost all of its usefulness when its owner shed his mortal shell? What was this intimate bond between the brace and this grave's inhabitant that compelled the deceased's loved ones to bury him wearing this earthly contraption?

The answer can start to be unravelled by the stone that lay above these skeletal remains. The stone reveals that the individual's name was Timothy Cratchit, son of Robert. The inhabitant of this forgotten London grave was Tiny Tim, son of Bob Cratchit, of Dickensian Christmas lore. The grave marker reads "In memory, Timothy Cratchit, 1839-1884. Beloved Husband of Julia, Father of Robert, and Son of Robert and Martha".

We learn that Timothy Cratchit did not die as a youth but, rather, died as an adult after being married and becoming a father himself. These facts are merely clues to the real lesson that the British novelist Charles Dickens was trying to teach the 19th century society in which he lived. This lost lesson of Tiny Tim is just as appropriate today as it was a century and a half ago.

This chapter examines and gives "rise the Ghost of an Idea [2]" which has been lost for the past century. It is the two-fold message which Dickens delivers through his character Tiny Tim. It is a call, on one level, for society to provide universal healthcare provisions for children while, on another level, it is a call to each individual to use whatever resources and/or power with which they are imbued to champion the cause of children's healthcare on a more personal level.

CHARLES DICKENS

Charles Dickens was born on February 7, 1812 to John and Elizabeth Dickens. Many of his childhood experiences influenced both his writings and his penchant for social advocacy. Dickens' early life was not easy. The family moved from one neighborhood to another until his father was put into a debtor's prison. Most of the family, with the exception of Charles, went to live with the father in prison. Dickens, 12, was forced to work at a blacking warehouse until his grandmother died and left enough of an inheritance for the father to be released from prison [3]. While working at the warehouse, Dickens often suffered from fever and spasms [3].

Dickens had an intense interest in the many facets of the human condition. This was especially true of the many medical maladies which were ever-present in London during his lifetime. Among Dickens' Victorian colleagues it was standard practice to invent maladies with inconsistent symptoms [4]. This was definitely not true of Dickens. Dickens made regular visits to hospitals to meet and observe the sick [5-7]. He was also a regular reader of The Lancet [5].

Dickens died of a cerebral hemorrhage at the age of 58 [8]. His magnificent works, filled with such vivid imagery of Victorian London, continue to delight and enthrall readers today. The British Medical Journal stated, upon his death, "What a gain it would have been to physic if one so keen to observe and so facile to describe had devoted his powers to the medical art [9]."

POTT'S DISEASE

Pott's Disease is tuberculosis of the spine [10]. The most commonly affected areas of the spine are the lower thoracic and upper lumbar vertebrae [11]. It was first described by Sir Percivall Pott (1714-1788). Most of the cases occur in children between 3 and 10 years of age. Symptoms in children include pain, stiffness in the back, gradual wasting, fevers and fatigue [1]. If left untreated, death will follow when the bone infection leaks into the spinal cord and brain causing meningitis [1].

TB of the spine must be differentiated from 'compression fractures'. This can be done by the use of an MRI scan. A biopsy of the spinal lesion, in those patients with Pott's Disease, will reveal *Mycobacterium tuberculosis* [12]. Samples were taken from the spine of the remains found in the grave of Timothy Cratchit. The

Microbiology Research Institute of Cambridge tested these samples by polymerase chain reaction. They tested positive for *Mycobacterium tuberculosis* [1].

Today, proper diagnosis of Pott's Disease along with anti-tuberculosis treatment will result in a cure [12]. Even in the days of Dickens, patients with Pott's Disease were occasionally seen to experience a remission [1] particularly if proper rest and bracing were provided.

DICKENS' HIDDEN MESSAGE

Charles Dickens frequently placed veiled messages in his work. Dickens was, in addition to being probably the greatest novelist in the history of the English language, a master observer, a champion of children, and a social reformer. He was also many years ahead of his time. 'The Lost Message of Tiny Tim' encompasses all the aforementioned attributes of Dickens. This message is not hidden but as in so many cases, society can not see what is plainly visible and thus, the message has become lost.

Through the decades 'A Christmas Carol' has been retold a countless number of times. Each rendition progressively degrading Dickens' original masterpiece and thus, further obscuring his message which is embodied in the persona of Tiny Tim. The message of Dickens is two-fold. Dickens calls for society to provide universal access to healthcare for children regardless of the financial status into which they were born. It is a call to the influential individuals of society- the lawmakers, the leaders of the healthcare professions and those special individuals of society whose voices carry much weight. It is a call to enact change on a societal level and to reach down and touch the lives of each and every- "God bless us, every one" [1]- child in society. Dickens addressed the skeptics who stated that such reform would be impossible. Dickens represented this social reform in the transformation of the character Scrooge- "some people laughed to see the alteration in him but he let them laugh, and little heeded them; for he was wise enough to know that nothing ever happened on this globe, for good, at which some people did not have their fill of laughter in the outset, and knowing that such as these would be blind anyway, he thought it quite as well that they should wrinkle up their eyes by grins as have the malady in less attractive forms. His own heart laughed: and that was quite enough for him [1]."

The second part of Dickens' 'lost message of Tiny Tim' is that in order to relieve some of the suffering of children, one needs not be a world-renowned novelist, a judge, a politician, a mogul, or a tycoon. Rather, as individuals we can affect a change in the life of a child whom we may encounter in our everyday life.

Scrooge's transformation is an integral part of 'the lost message of Tiny Tim'. Scrooge underwent his own personal transformation when he grasped the message embodied by the small disabled child. Scrooge realized the value and preciousness of the life and well-being of the child as being "as good as gold, and better [1]." He realized that the child did not have to die- it was not a predestined fact. He understood that by his actions alone, the child's life could be saved. Dickens explicitly states that Tiny Tim did not die- "Scrooge was better than his word. He did it all and infinitely more; and to Tiny Tim, who did not die, he was a second father [1]." By this statement, Dickens illustrates the power and possibility of the individual.

REFERENCES

[1]   Callahan CW. Construction crew discovers grave of "Tiny Tim". The Journal of Infectious Diseases 1997; 176: 1652-1654.
[2]   Dickens CA. A Christmas Carol and other holiday tales. Ann Arbor; Border Classics, 2003.
[3]   Vittum HE. Charles Dickens: a biographical sketch. New York; Bantam Dell, 1965.
[4]   Markel H. Charles Dickens and the art of medicine. Ann Intern Med 1984; 101: 408-411.
[5]   Markel H. Charles Dickens' work to help establish Great Ormond Street Hospital, London. Lancet 1999; 354: 673-675.
[6]   Poynten FNL. Thomas Southwood Smith- The man. Proc R Soc Med 1962; 55: 381-392.
[7]   Fielding KJ, ed. The Speeches of Charles Dickens. Oxford: Clarendon Press, 1960; 40-43, 222-225, 246-253.
[8]   Schoffer KL, O'Sullivan JD. Charles Dickens: the man, medicine, and movement disorders. Journal of Clinical Neuroscience 2006; 13(9): 898-901.
[9]   Wood J. Passion and pathology in Victorian fiction (1st ed.), New York; Oxford University Press; 2001.

[10] Bouvresse S, Chiras J, Bricaire F, Bossi P. Pott's disease occurring after percutaneous vertebroplasty: an unusual illustration of the principle of locus minoris resistentiae. Journal of Infection 2006; 53(6): e251-e253.

[11] British Society for Antimicrobial Chemotherapy. Pott's Disease. Accessed on March 26, 2011. Available at www.bsac.org.uk/pyxls/Bone%20and%20joint/Potts%/20disease? Potts%/20disease/Potts%20disease.htm.

[12] Dass B, Puet TA, Watanakunakorn C. Tuberculosis of the spine (Pott's Disease) presenting as 'compression fractures.' Spinal Cord 2002; 40(11): 604-608.

| CHAPTER 9 |

The Cancer of President U.S. Grant

Abstract: This chapter analyzes the oral squamous cell carcinoma of American Civil War hero Ulysses Grant. Today, the deleterious effects of the use of alcohol and tobacco are well documented and many forms of oral cancer can now be treated very successfully if diagnosed at an early stage. Such was not the case in the nineteenth century. Grant's case illustrates both the need for early detection of head and neck cancers and the importance of the public understanding the harmful effects of tobacco and alcohol.

Keywords: American Civil War, biopsy, epithelioma, exophytic, hypoepiglottic ligament, leukoplakia, lymph nodes, nicotine, optical diagnosis, oral cancer, oral medicine, photodynamic diagnosis, squamous cell carcinoma, oral pathology.

INTRODUCTION

Ulysses Grant rose from a rather inauspicious start in his military career to becoming the symbol of the victorious Union states during the war for Southern independence. On Good Friday in 1865 it was thrust upon his shoulders to become the champion of the now deceased President Lincoln's conciliatory and generous Reconstruction plans. The powerful General from West Point would show tolerance, mercy, and kindness towards his former Southern adversaries who fought a valiant yet bloody four year battle.

Grant would later trade in the title 'General-in-Chief' for 'Commander-in-Chief' as he and his family took up residence in the White House for two terms. Unfortunately, for Grant, life did not show him the mercy in the years following his presidency that he had shown towards the Southern states and their leaders. His final years were filled with unscrupulous business partners and predatory publishers who led to his financial ruin. Grant would be saved, financially, by his friend, Mark Twain, who convinced the General to let Twain's new publishing company publish his memoirs. This was a godsend financially yet, the General still had one final battle to fight- this time against oral squamous cell carcinoma.

Historian Allan Nevins notes that "his one vice, when he entered the White House, was tobacco. He reeked with it; his cigars were black, rank and poisonous; he consumed them in huge quantities." This tobacco habit had gripped Grant since the Mexican War in the 1840's [1]. The amount and frequency of Grant's alcohol use is subject to much historical debate. Many have, most probably erroneously, portrayed Grant as an alcoholic. Grant did occasionally drink alcohol but, there are no reliable witnesses that had ever stated that Grant was ever inebriated during the Civil War [2]. The tag of being an alcoholic was most likely placed on him by the gossip and rumors of jealous Union generals.

HIRAM ULYSSES GRANT

On April 27, 1822 a ten and three-quarters pounds baby boy was born at Point Pleasant, Ohio. This infant would eventually rise to prominence as a military hero in the Western Theater of Operations during the American Civil War. The father, Jesse Root Grant, and the mother, Hannah Simpson Grant, struggled to find a suitable name for their newborn son. The father favored Hiram; the maternal grandparents suggested Ulysses and the mother wanted to name her son Albert Gallatin in honor of Jefferson's Secretary of the Treasury and founder of New York University. The child was eventually named Hiram Ulysses Grant partly hinting at the heroic stature the child would attain later in life [3].

Grant's ancestral roots lay in the early colonial land of the East. In 1630, Matthew Grant arrived in the Massachusetts Bay Colony. Successive generations creeped slowly westward in the new, uncharted land from the Connecticut River to Pennsylvania to Kentucky and, eventually, to Ohio. Grant was born with the blood of military heroes running through his veins. His forefathers fought the first battles of the brave, new nation. One of his great-grandfathers was killed in action during the French and Indian War while another fought with Washington during the Revolutionary War. His grandfather fought at Bunker Hill [3, 4].

In 1839, at seventeen-years-old, Grant entered the United States Military Academy at West Point much to his displeasure. Upon arrival at West Point, a serendipitous clerical error presented itself. On the list of new cadets there was no sign of a Hiram U. Grant. Rather, his name was listed as U.S. Grant. Grant did not complain about the error in his name. Henceforward, this would be the name of the future hero of the nation.

Grant proved to be a great horseman at West Point but, did not show much promise for a successful military career. Upon graduation from West Point, Grant married his West Point roommate's sister, Julia Dent. He then served in the military during the Mexican War, which he thought was an unjust war, and later, was assigned to Fort Vancouver and, finally, a post in California. Grant resigned from the Army on April 11, 1854.

Grant tried his hand at business during this interbellum period. He had little success and reenlisted in the Army in 1861 at the start of the Civil War. His victories in the Western Theater coupled with a series of inept Union commanders garnered Grant much praise from President Lincoln leading to his appointment as commander of the Union Army culminating with his acceptance of General Robert E. Lee's surrender in 1865. The immense popularity and gratitude showered upon the 'Hero of Appomattox' translated into two terms in the White House. However, Grant's post-presidential years were not kind to him. He suffered through financial ruin and eventually passed away in 1885 from the effects of oral squamous cell carcinoma.

ORAL SQUAMOUS CELL CARCINOMA

Squamous cell carcinoma is the most common form of either oral or pharyngeal carcinoma [5]. Oral squamous cell carcinoma has, until recently, been found primarily in elderly men and has been associated with excessive alcohol and tobacco use [6].

The chief risk factors for oral squamous cell carcinoma continue to be smoking and alcohol use with the combination of heavy smoking and alcohol abuse increasing the risk of developing this cancer by 100 times in women and 38 times in men [5]. Other risk factors include chewing tobacco, chronic irritation, betel quid, the oral human papillomavirus, and the overuse of mouthwash [5, 7].

An individual's predilection to be dependent on alcohol seems to be linked to their dependence on tobacco products. Almost 80% of individuals who are dependent on alcohol have been reported to smoke cigarettes [8]. In addition, the nicotine dependence of smokers appears to be more severe in those individuals who also have a history of alcohol dependence [9]. It has also been documented that the risk for a second primary tumor is increased in those individuals with a previous upper aerodigestive tract tumor [5, 10].

The floor of the mouth or the lateral and ventral surfaces of the tongue are the sites of 40% of oral squamous cell carcinomas. 38% occur on the lower lip which are usually related to exposure to the sun. 11% begin in the tonsillar area and the palate [5].

It is imperative that all individuals receive proper and thorough oral examinations and head/neck examinations. This will increase the chance of a potentially cancerous lesion being detected early. This, in turn, will lead to an increased chance of survival. Oral squamous cell carcinoma lesions may appear to be areas of erythroplakia or leukoplakia. They may be exophytic or ulcerated, indurated or firm with a rolled border. Carcinoma in the tonsillar region might present with an asymmetric swelling, sore throat, and pain radiating to the ipsilateral ear [5].

Today, there are many modern means and methods of oral cytology for oral squamous cell carcinoma. One such method is DNA image cytometry. This method measures DNA ploidy. It compares Feulgen dye-stained cytologic samples with normal epithelial cells. By examining these samples in such a manner the malignancy of oral mucosal cells can be determined [6]. It has been shown that the nuclear DNA content of oral leukoplakia cells are able to be used to predict the oral epithelial dysplasia up to 5 years before a diagnosis may be made histologically [11].

Another diagnostic method is photodynamic diagnosis. This method uses 5-aminolevulinic acid. It is administered either systemically or applied topically to the oral mucosa and facial skin [6]. It has been demonstrated to have a sensitivity of 83-90% and a specificity of 79-89% [12].

Other methods of diagnosis include biopsy, endoscopy, cytomorphometry, optical diagnosis, and chest x-ray and CT scan of the head and neck region.

GRANT'S FINAL BATTLE

A tobacco habit had gripped Grant since the Mexican War in the 1840's. The amount and frequency of Grant's alcohol use is subject to much historical debate. Many have, most probably erroneously, portrayed Grant as an alcoholic. Grant probably drank alcohol most frequently during his early years in the army when he was assigned to lonely, distant outposts.

While vacationing in early June of 1884 in the seaside resort town of Long Branch, New Jersey Grant bit into a peach. He immediately felt a sting in his throat. This was the first sign of Grant's cancer. It is postulated that what he was feeling was the tumor pushing through the hypoepiglottic ligament [13]. Dr. Jacob Mendez Da Costa was visiting next door at the time and urged him to see Dr. Fordyce Barker in New York. Unfortunately, Grant declined to have the lesion examined further until October.

Grant started to develop some soreness in the right tonsillar region and by October one of the lymph nodes located under the angle of the mandible on the right side had become enlarged and an ulceration was present at the base of the right tonsillar pillar. At this time, Dr. John Douglas, an associate of Dr. Barker and an acquaintance of the former president from over twenty years prior at Fort Donelson, took over the care of Grant's unknown ailment. On October 22, 1884 at 11 a.m. Dr. Douglas examined Grant and found his soft palate to be "inflamed, of a dark, deep congestive hue, a scaly squamous inflammation strongly suggestive of serious epithelial trouble." Grant's tongue was also swollen on the right side. Grant could see the concern in his doctor's face and asked him very simply, "Is it cancer?" Dr. Douglas avoided telling Grant the truth [14].

On February 18, 1885 a biopsy was performed by one of Dr. Barker's surgical associates, Dr. F.C. Riley, who gave the specimen to the pathologist, Dr. George R. Elliott. Dr. Elliott gave a diagnosis of epithelioma or, in modern terms, squamous carcinoma. Microscopic observation revealed irregularly shaped epithelial cells which had formed into concentric globes indicating rapid growth and blood vessels with decidedly thick walls.

In early April, Grant was suffering tremendously. He had a falling pulse, increased salivation, and a spasmodic cough. He received atropine at night, five drops of digitalis every 5 hours, and morphine injections [15].

On April 7, Grant hemorrhaged severely but, subsequently, made a dramatic improvement which allowed him to resume work on his memoirs. The improvement was due to a large portion of the tumor sloughing off thus making it easier for Grant to breathe. Each night he would sleep sitting up between two leather chairs as he feared choking to death. At this point Grant was receiving morphine and cocaine for his pain. On June 16, 1885 Grant moved to the peaceful and serene setting of Mt. McGregor, New York to spend his final days [3].

As Grant spent his last days at Mt. McGregor, he was cognizant that the end of his final earthly battle approached. The final moments of the great General's life were not marked by a heroic cavalry charge, the laying down of arms, or the unfurling of flags. Rather, Grant simply placed a farewell note in the pocket of his bathrobe to be found after his passing by his wife- "I bid you a final farewell, until we meet in another and, I trust, better world".

REFERENCES

[1]   Bunting J. Ulysses S. Grant: The American Presidents Series: The 18th President, 1869-1877, New York: Times Books, 2004.
[2]   Meives D. Little known facts about Ulysses S. Grant. Available at: http://faculty.css.edu/mkelsey/usgrant/facts.html. Accessed 3/15/11.
[3]   Smith JE. Grant, New York: Simon and Schuster Paperbacks, 2001.
[4]   Grant US. The Complete Personal Memoirs of Ulysses S. Grant, United States of America: Seven Treasures Publications, 2010.
[5]   The Merck Manual. Oral squamous cell carcinoma. Accessed on 8/24/12. Available at: www.merckmanuals.com/professional/ear_nose_and_throat_disorders_and_neck/oral_squamous_cell/tumors_of_the_head_carcinoma.html
[6]   Zygogianni AG, Kyrgias G, Karakitsos P, *et al*. Oral squamous cell cancer: early detection and the role of alcohol and smoking. Head Neck Oncol. 2011; 3: 2.
[7]   Shiboski CH, Schmidt BL, Jordan RC. Tongue and tonsil carcinoma: increasing trends in the US population ages 20-44 years. Cancer. 2005; 103(9): 1843-1849.
[8]   Kohn CS, Tsoh, JY, Weisner CM. Changes in smoking status among substance abusers: baseline characteristics and abstinence from alcohol and drugs at 12-month follow-up. Drug Alcohol Depend. 2003; 69: 61-71.

[9]   Marks JL, Hill EM, Pomerleau CS, Mudd SA, Blow FC. Nicotine dependence and withdrawal in alcoholic and nonalcoholic ever-smokers. J Subst Abuse Treat 1997; 14: 521-527.

[10]   Do KA, Johnson MM, Doherty DA, *et al*. Second primary tumors in patients with upper aerodigestive tract cancers: joint effects of smoking and alcohol (United States) Cancer Causes Control. 2003; 14: 131-138.

[11]   Sudbo J, Kildal W, Risberg B, Koppang HS, Danielsen HE, Reith A. DNA content as a prognostic marker in patients with oral leukoplakia. N Eng J Med 2001; 344: 1270-1278.

[12]   Sharwani A, Jerjes W, Salih V, *et al*. Fluoresence spectroscopy combined with 5-aminolevulinic acid-induced protoporphyrin IX fluorescence in detecting oral premalignancy. J Photochem Photobiol B. 2006; 83: 27-33.

[13]   Sharrer T. What's in Grant's tumor? Available at: http:// www.thehistorychannelclub. com/articles/articletype/articleview/articleid/136/whats-in- grants-tumor. Accessed on 3/15/11.

[14]   Steckler RM, Shedd DP. General Grant: his physicians and his cancer. Am J Surg 1976 Oct; 132(4): 508-514.

[15]   Shrady GF. The surgical and pathological aspects of General Grant's case. Medical Record 28: 121, 1885.

CHAPTER 10

The Implications of the Hemophilia of Queen Victoria

Abstract: Queen Victoria reigned over Great Britain from 1840 to 1901. Her marriage to Albert resulted in nine offspring. These children later married into various royal families of Europe bringing with them the genetic trait for hemophilia. Hemophilia is a hereditary blood disorder in which the blood does not clot in the usual manner. The fact that Victoria was a carrier for hemophilia raises the logical question of why there were no signs of hemophilia in any of her male ancestors.

Keywords: Blood disorder, Christmas Disease, clot, Eugenie, fibrinolysis, genetics, hemophilia, hereditary, Leopold, Rasputin, reign, the royal disease, throne.

QUEEN VICTORIA

Victoria, the only daughter of Edward, Duke of Kent (fourth son of George III), was born on May 24, 1819 at Kensington Palace in London, England [1]. Her mother, Victoria Maria Louisa of Saxe-Coburg, was the sister of Leopold, King of the Belgians. She served as Queen of the United Kingdom of Great Britain and Ireland from 1837 to 1901 and as Empress of India from 1876 until her death [2]. Victoria would reign through many decades but, it would not be until a history lesson at age ten that she would discover that she would one day be the ruler of the British empire. The startled child reacted by making a promise to her governess-"I will be good" [2].

Victoria's father died shortly after her birth. Victoria became heir to the throne because her three uncles had no legitimate offspring who survived infancy. This is especially astonishing considering that Victoria's grandfather, King George III, had 15 children [2].

Her childhood was simple and unhappy as it was controlled by her mother's advisor, Sir John Conroy. There has been much speculation by many historians that Conroy was actually Victoria's biological father. I believe it highly unlikely that Conroy was Victoria's father as he led a very physically active life while never exhibiting any signs of hemophilia. This does not preclude another individual, other than the Duke of Kent, to have fathered Victoria. Upon the death of William IV, Victoria ascended to the throne in 1837 at the age of 18 [1].

The early years of Victoria's reign were greatly influenced by her first prime minister, Lord Melbourne. Melbourne gave her confidence and sound advice. Melbourne resigned from office in May of 1839. He resumed his office after his successor Robert Peel had a disagreement with Victoria over what became known as "the bedchamber crisis" [2].

On February 10, 1840 Queen Victoria married her cousin, Prince Albert of Saxe-Coburg and Gotha. This marriage produced children both quickly and often. This is where the tragic story of 'the royal disease', hemophilia, begins. The couple's first child was Victoria who was born later in 1840. 18 years later she married the crown prince of Prussia. The other children were the Prince of Wales (later Edward   VII), Princess Alice, Prince Alfred, Princess Helena, Princess Louise, Prince Arthur, Prince Leopold, and Princess Beatrice [2]. These children married into many of the royal families of Europe bringing the genetic trait for hemophilia with them.

When Albert died in 1861, Victoria sank into depression and would wear black for the remainder of her reign to memorialize him [1].

Many political reforms occurred during Victoria's reign which moved much power away from the monarch and into the hands of the people [3]. Victoria was much admired and reigned over a period of time which also saw huge advances in technology, culture, and science.

The end of Victoria's reign was overshadowed by the Boer War in South Africa during which she remained steadfast in her belief in British military invincibility-"We are not interested in the possibilities of defeat; they do not exist."

The longest reigning British monarch died on January 22, 1901 and is buried, next to Albert, at Windsor, in the Frogmore Royal Mausoleum.

HEMOPHILIA

Hemophilia is a rare hereditary bleeding disorder in which the blood does not clot in a normal manner at the site of a wound or injury. There are two main types of inherited hemophilia- Type A and Type B (Christmas Disease). There is a deficiency of Factor VIII in Type A while there is a deficiency in Factor IX in Type B [4]. The gene for hemophilia is located on the x chromosome. They are clinically similar x-linked recessive disorders [5]. Hemophilia is almost always found exclusively in males while females can be carriers and pass it down to their offspring [6]. Approximately 9 out of 10 individuals who have hemophilia have Type A. There is also a non-inherited hemophilia whereby the body starts to attack and destroy its own clotting factors. This type is very rare [6]. The incidence of Type A is 1/5,000 live male births while the incidence of Type B is 1/300,000 live male births [7]. Individuals with Hemophilia A demonstrate bleeding tendencies which are not always predicted by their Factor VIII level. It has been suggested that bleeding in hemophilia is not only due to defective prothrombin activation but also aberrant fibrinolysis [7].

Hemophilia may lead to joint swelling that can lead to damage or swelling in the muscle; bleeding in the head and sometimes in the brain which can lead to brain damage; damage to other organs; and death which can occur if bleeding can not be stopped or if bleeding occurs in a vital organ (*i.e.,* brain) [8].

Presently there are 141 federally-funded treatment centers and programs across the United States which provide comprehensive care for the whole individual and the family. As a result, individuals with bleeding disorders have become more independent and productive with an improved quality of life [9].

THE ROYAL DISEASE

Queen Victoria was a carrier of the gene for hemophilia and eventually passed it down to the royal families of Germany, Russia, and Spain [10, 11]. Prince Leopold was born on April 7, 1853. His birth marked the first instance of hemophilia in the British royal family. Leopold was Victoria and Albert's eighth child and fourth son. Prior to Leopold, no occurrence of hemophilia in the royal family had been known. This is extremely important as one must thus conclude that a mutation must have occurred as an extremely rare *de novo* point mutation in the sperm of Queen Victoria's father, Edward Augustus, Duke of Kent [12]. Otherwise, the only other scientific explanation as to the origin of Victoria's recessive trait is that Queen Victoria's birth was of an illegitimate nature. The Royal Society of Medicine has investigated seventeen generations of the family on Queen Victoria's mother's side. Not one had hemophilia [13].

The first written allusion to the hemophilia of the British royal family was in the British Medical Journal of February 8, 1868. It stated that His Royal Highness Prince Leopold, "who had previously been in full health and activity, has been suffering during the last week from severe accidental haemorrhage. The Prince was reduced to a state of extreme and dangerous exhaustion by the loss of blood, but has since greatly recovered and has regained his strength [14]." Leopold was the only son of Victoria to suffer from hemophilia. However, Victoria's youngest child, Beatrice, gave birth to Eugenie who was a carrier and later married King Alonso XIII of Spain [15-18]. The couple had five sons. Four out of the five suffered from hemophilia. The Spanish royal family was discredited as they had the legacy of heirs disinherited on medical grounds [13, 14].

Alice, Queen Victoria's third child, passed hemophilia to the German and Russian imperial families. Alice had two daughters- Irene and Alix. Irene married Prince Henry of Prussia, her first cousin. The couple had two hemophiliac sons. Alix married Tsar Nikolas II of the Russian Imperial family. Their fifth child was finally the long-awaited son, Alexis, heir to the Russian throne. It was obvious from a very early age that Alexis suffered from hemophilia. His father became preoccupied with Alexis's illness and the affairs of the state deteriorated. The family turned to a spiritualist, Rasputin, who seemed to be able to relieve the boy's suffering. The grateful family gave Rasputin unlimited trust. These factors led to the Russian Revolution and the eventual execution of the entire Russian royal family [12].

The role of hemophilia in the politics and history of the 19th and 20th centuries is obvious. The source of the royal disease, Victoria, is also obvious. Victoria's cursed royal blood flowed through the palaces and royal courts of Europe. Not so obvious is the source of Victoria's own possession of the genetic code for hemophilia. Was it truly a rare spontaneous mutation? Was it the result of Victoria's mother's purported relationship with John Conroy? Or, more likely, another man other than her husband or Conroy? At the present time that is all still up for speculation but it could be solved relatively easily with a simple kinship test. However, for this to occur certain royal individuals must realize that science and history share one singular goal- the truth- and all the implications that the truth does hold.

REFERENCES

[1]   The British Monarchy. Accessed on 8/5/12. Available at: www.royal.gov.uk/historyofthem onarchy/kingsandqueensoftheunitedkingdom/thehanoverians/victoria.aspx.

[2]   Victoria. Accessed on 8/20/12. Available at: www.spartacus.schoolast.co.uk/ prvictoria. htm.

[3]   PBS. Accessed on 8/6/12. Available at: http://www.biography.com/people/queen- victoria= 951835.

[4]   The Cleveland Clinic. Hemophilia. Accessed on 3/31/11. Available at: http:// my.clevelandclinic.org/disorders/hemophilia/hiC_what_is_hemophilia.aspx.

[5]   Wilker SC, Singh A, Ellis FJ. Recurrent bleeding following traumatic hyphema due to mild hemophilia B (Christmas disease). Journal of American Association for Pediatric Ophthalmology and Strabismus 2007; 11(6): 622-623.

[6]   National Heart, Lung and Blood Institute. What causes hemophilia? Accessed on 3/31/11. Available at: http://www.nhlbi.nih.gov/health/dci/Diseases/hemophilia/ hemophilia_causes. html.

[7]   Gomez-Moreno G, Cutando-Soriano A, Arana C, Scully C. Hereditary blood coagulation disorders: management and dental treatment. J Dent Res 2005; 84(11): 978-985.

[8]   Foley JH, Nesheim ME, Rivard GE, Brummel-Ziedins KE. Thrombin activable fibrinolysis inhibitor activation and bleeding in haemophilia A. Haemophilia. Epud ahead of print 20 Sep 2011.

[9]   Centers for Disease Control and Prevention. Hemophilia. Accessed on 3/31/11. Available at: http://www.cdc.gov/ncbddd/hemophilia/facts.html.

[10]   Aronova-Tiuntseva Y, Herreid CF. Hemophilia: "The Royal Disease". Accessed on 3/30/11. Available at: http://www.sciencecases.org/hemo/hemo.asp.

[11]   Kumar JN, Kumar RA, Varadarajan R, Sharma N. Specialty dentistry for the hemophiliac: is there a protocol in place? Indian J Dent Res 2007; 18: 48-54.

[12]   Haemophilia in the descendants of Queen Victoria. Accessed on 3/30/11. Available at: http://www.englishmonarchs.co.uk/haemophilia.html.

[13]   The Daily Mail. Accessed on 3/30/11. Available at: http://www.dailymail.co.uk/femail/ article-1158993/were-Queen-Victoria-Price-Albert-illegitimate.html.

[14]   British Medical Journal. Article. Br Med J 1868; 1: 122.

[15]   Aronova-Tiuntseva Y, Herreid CF. Hemophilia: "The Royal Disease". Accessed on 4/4/11. Availanle at: http://www.sciencecases.org/hemo/hemo.pdf.
[16]   Kingston HM. Autumn Books. Br Med J 1995; 311(7012): 1106.
[17]   Potts DM, Potts WTW, Sutton A. Queen Victoria's gene: haemophilia and the royal family 1995; Great Britain: Sutton Publishing Limited.
[18]   Lombard J. Root canal hemorrhages in endodontics: a preventive solution. Chir Dent Fr 1976; 46: 45-51.

CHAPTER 11

The Hypertension of President Franklin Delano Roosevelt

Abstract: Franklin Roosevelt was born into an aristocratic American family. His childhood was one of wealth and privilege. He had very little in common with the trials and tribulations of the average American youth. He later became America's only four-term president and served in that capacity during a particularly tumultuous period of American history. President Roosevelt suffered from hypertension. His blood pressure rose steadily as he led the nation through the Great Depression and World War II. The medical professionals of Roosevelt's era did not have a very thorough understanding of hypertension. Fortunately, there are many effective medications available today for those who are hypertensive. There has been considerable research performed since the 1940's which has greatly expanded the medical community's knowledge of hypertension and its effects.

Keywords: Diastolic, diet, FDR, high blood pressure, hypertension, hypertensive crisis, prehypertension, stage 1 hypertension, stage 2 hypertension, systolic, The Great Depression, thiazide diuretics, Warm Springs, World War II.

PRESIDENT FRANKLIN ROOSEVELT

Franklin Delano Roosevelt was born on January 30, 1882 at 8:45 in the evening. James and Sara Roosevelt were overjoyed at the arrival of their ten pound baby boy. The couple named the child in honor of Sara's favorite uncle, Franklin Delano. The wealthy couple surely had great aspirations for their son but, even the proud parents could not have imagined the life that lay ahead for their son. This infant eventually become the only four-term president of the United States and lead the nation through the bleak days of the Great Depression and the nightmares of World War II. He would become beloved by his countrymen, feared by his enemies, and known to all simply as FDR [1].

Young Franklin was born into one of the wealthiest families in America. The Roosevelt Family was truly American aristocracy. FDR grew up in the beautiful family house, Springwood, in Hyde Park, New York. Springwood provided the family with beautiful views of the majestic Hudson River. The house can still be visited today as it is maintained as a unit of the National Parks System.

Roosevelt became paralyzed from the waist down from what was diagnosed as being polio. It is thought that he contracted a virus while visiting a Boy Scout encampment at Bear Mountain, New York on July 28, 1921. He became paralyzed from the waist down and never walked again without the aid of canes, crutches or braces. Out of respect, the press never published photographs displaying his disability.

THE PRESIDENT'S SACRIFICE

The four terms of FDR's presidency were filled with much grief, angst, and turmoil for Americans. The same was true for people throughout the world. The aristocratically born FDR personally felt the suffering of the people. It took a fatal toll on his health. As the stresses rose, so did the President's blood pressure. Much can be learned from the study of FDR's untreated hypertension. One thing that is certain is that FDR sacrificed his life to lead the free people of the world out of the grips of tyrannical leaders.

FDR was campaigning for his first term as president of the United States in 1931. At that time he released his medical records. It is apparent that FDR was already suffering from hypertension with a reading of 140/100. FDR won the election and selected Admiral Ross McIntire to be his personal physician. Admiral McIntire was an ear, nose, and throat specialist [2].

The stress of the immense workload and the thousands of miles of travel began to take a toll on FDR's health. This could be seen by his blood pressure measurements. In 1937, at the beginning of his second term, Roosevelt's systolic reached 169 (169/98) [2]. In 1940, FDR gave up his daily exercise of swimming in the White House pool [1]. The following year, 1941, saw a dramatic deterioration in both the President's health and relations with Japan. His blood pressure was 188/105 on February 27, 1941. However, there were no outward signs of hypertension [2] at this point.

The next four years saw brutal fighting in Europe and the Pacific. Roosevelt continued to lead the free world bravely onward towards victory as his own health steadily declined. Roosevelt started experiencing headaches in January of 1944 and sometimes fell asleep during conversations [3]. His family grew concerned. Anna, FDR's daughter, was losing faith in her father's physician.

On March 27, 1944 Roosevelt was brought to Bethesda Naval Hospital. A lieutenant commander in the Naval Reserve, Dr. Howard G. Bruenn, examined FDR. He was ordered by Admiral McIntire to report his findings to him while revealing nothing to the President [1]. Bruenn found FDR to have heart disease, bronchitis, left ventricular cardiac failure and hypertension (186/108) [4]. He felt that if FDR did not receive proper medical attention he would be dead within a year [1]. These findings were not told to FDR. By the next month, April 1944, FDR's fate was sealed with a blood pressure of 210/120.

The end finally came on April 12, 1945 as FDR posed for a portrait by artist Elizabeth Shoumatoff. Suddenly FDR raised his left hand to his temple, squeezed his forehead and stated that he had a terrible headache. Subsequently, he lost consciousness. Dr. Bruenn was by the President's side and took his blood pressure one last time. It was 300/190. FDR had suffered a fatal brain hemorrhage and was declared dead two hours later, at 3:45 p.m., by Dr. Bruenn [2].

HYPERTENSION

Fortunately, there have been many pharmaceutical discoveries since the time of FDR which help regulate an individual's blood pressure. The major types of medications for hypertension are thiazide diuretics, beta blockers, angiotensin-converting enzyme inhibitors, calcium channel blockers, renin inhibitors, alpha blockers, alpha-beta blockers, central acting agents, and non-thiazide diuretic drugs [3-5].

Some possible complications of hypertensive treatment include orthostatic hypotension [6, 7], xerostomia [6, 8], gingival overgrowth [6, 9-12], lichenoid reations [6, 7, 13-16], scalded mouth syndrome [6, 17], potential drug interactions [6, 18-20], and the prolonged use of nonsteroidal anti-inflammatory agents which may decrease the anti-hypertensive effectiveness of certain hypertension drugs [6, 21].

In the United States alone, between 50 million [22] and 65 million individuals [23] are affected by hypertension. It is the most common primary diagnosis in the United States [6]. It is known as a silent killer because only 30% of hypertensive individuals are aware that they have this condition [6, 24-26].

The blood pressure measurement consists of two numerical readings. The systolic is the measure of the pressure in the arteries when the heart muscle contracts and the diastolic is the pressure in the resting heart muscle [22]. There are five categories of blood pressure readings. They are normal, prehypertension, hypertension stage 1, hypertension stage 2, and hypertensive crisis [27].

There are certain lifestyle measures which people should follow to either avoid becoming hypertensive or to decrease the effects of hypertension. They are smoking cessation [23], maintaining ideal body weight [6, 23, 28, 29], exercise [6, 23, 30, 31], decrease stress and anger [23], sodium reduction [6, 23, 31-33], taking medications properly [23], eating many fruits, vegetables, and low-fat dairy products [6, 32], avoiding alcohol [6, 23, 33], eating foods rich in potassium [23], and having proper medical care [23].

It is known that hypertension is a major risk factor for stroke, kidney disease, heart attack, and heart failure, However, proper hypertensive therapy has been demonstrated to decrease the incidence of myocardial infarction by up to 25%, heart failure by more than 50%, and stroke by up to 40 % [6, 34].

CONCLUSION

President Roosevelt spent much time towards the end of his life at a small cottage retreat in Warm Springs, Georgia because of his paralytic disability. The Warm Springs Foundation was founded and it eventually became The March of Dimes Association. Through the wonderful work of this organization a cure for polio was eventually discovered [35].

Some historians still debate as to whether FDR was actually aware of his deadly blood pressure readings. It is very obvious that Roosevelt was aware of his declining health and how it would eventually end for him. He truly sacrificed himself for the good of the nation and the world.

The medical community's knowledge of hypertension and its effects certainly was in its infancy in the 1940's. However, Admiral McIntire was well aware of the damage that was being done to the President. Within hours after FDR's death, all of Roosevelt's medical records disappeared from a locked safe at Bethesda Naval Hospital. To this day these records have not been recovered.

REFERENCES

[1]   Smith JE. FDR 440, 602, 603 and n, 604, 606, 628, 635, 672n9 (New York: Random House Trade Paperbacks, 2007).
[2]   U.S. News & World Report. A change of heart: FDR's death shows how much we've learned about the heart. 2010. Available at: http://health.usnews.com/usnews/health/articles/050214/14heart_print.htm.
[3]   Doctor Zebra. Franklin Roosevelt. 2010. Available at: http://www.doctorzebra.com/prez/t32.htm.
[4]   Health Media Lab. Franklin Delano Roosevelt (1933-1945): The dying president. 2010. Available at: http://www.healthmedialab.com/html/president/roosevelt.html.
[5]   Mayo Clinic. High blood pressure (hypertension) treatment and drugs. 2010. Available at: http://www.mayoclinic.com/health/high-blood-pressure/DS00100?DSCTION=treatments%2Dand%2Ddrugs.
[6]   Herman WW, Konzelman JL, Prisant LM. New national guidelines on hypertension. J Am Dent Assoc 2004; 135(5): 576-584.
[7]   Little JW. The impact on dentistry of recent advances in the management of hypertension. Oral Surg Oral Med Oral Pathol Oral Radiol Endod 2000; 90: 591-599.
[8]   Navazesh M. How can oral health care providers determine if patients have dry mouth? JADA 2003; 134: 613-620.
[9]   Ellis JS, Seymour RA, Steele JG, Robertson P, Butler TJ, Thomason JM. Prevalence of gingival overgrowth induced by calcium channel blockers: a community-based study. J Periodontol 1999; 70(1): 63-67.
[10]   Prisant LM, Herman W. Calcium channel blocker induced gingival overgrowth. J Clin Hypertens 2002; 4(4): 310-311.
[11]   Miranda J, Brunet I, Roset P, Berini L, Farre M, Mendieta C. Prevalence and risk of gingival enlargement in patients with nifedipine. J Periodontol 2001; 72: 605-611.
[12]   Tavassoli S, Yamalik N, Caglayan G, Eratalay K. The Clinical effects of nifedipine on periodontal status. J Periodontol 1998; 69(2): 108-112.
[13]   Williams BG. Oral drug reaction to methyldopa: report of a case. Oral Surg Oral Med Oral Pathol 1983; 56: 375-377.

[14] Firth NA, Reade PC. Angiotensin-converting enzyme inhibitors implicated in oral mucosal lichenoid reactions. Oral Surg Oral Med Oral Pathol 1992; 74: 183-185.

[15] Riley CK, Terezhalmy GT. The patient with hypertension. Quintessence Int 2001; 32: 671-690.

[16] Robertson WD, Wray D. Ingestion of medication among patients with keratoses including lichen planus. Oral Surg Oral Med Oral Pathol 1992; 74: 183-185.

[17] Brown RS, Krakow AM, Douglas T, Choksi SK. 'Scalded mouth syndrome' caused by angiotensin converting enzyme inhibitors: two case reports. Oral Surg Oral Med Oral Pathol Oral Radiol Endod 1997; 83: 665-667.

[18] Bader JD, Bonito AJ, Shugars DA. A Systematic review of cardiovascular effects of epinephrine on hypertensive dental patients. Oral Surg Oral Med Oral Pathol Oral Radiol Endod 2002; 93: 647-653.

[19] Becker DE. The autonomic nervous system and related drugs in dental practice, part II: adrenergic agonists and antagonists. Compendium 1988; 9: 772-774, 776, 778-780.

[20] Sugimura M, Hirota Y, Shibutani T, *et al.* An electrocardiographic study of interactions between pindol and epinephrine contained in a local anesthetic solution. Anesth Prog 1995; 42(2): 29-35.

[21] Replogle K, Reader A, Nist R, Beck M, Weaver J, Meyers WJ. Cardiovascular effects of intraosseous injections of 2 percent lidocaine with 1: 100,000 epinephrine and 3 percent mepivicaine. JADA 1999; 130: 701-709.

[22] Hajjar I, Kotchen TA. Trends in prevalence, awareness, treatment, and control of hypertension in the United States, 1988-2000. JAMA 2003; 290(2): 199-206.

[23] Cleveland Clinic Miller Family Heart & Vascular Institute. Strategies to control high blood pressure. 2010. Available at: http://my.clevelandclinic.org/heart/prevention/htn/hpstrat.aspx.

[24] Vassan RS, Beiser A, Seshadri S, *et al.* Residual lifetime risk for developing hypertension in middle-aged women and men: The Framingham Heart Study. JAMA 2002; 287: 1003-1010.

[25] Chobanian AV, Bakris GL, Black HR, *et al.*: National Heart, Lung, and Blood Institute Joint National Committee on Prevention, Detection, Evaluation, and Treatment of High Blood Pressure; National High Blood Pressure Education program Coordinating Committee. The Seventh Report of the Joint National Committee on Prevention, Detection, Evaluation, and Treatment of High Blood Pressure: the JNC7 report (published correction appears in JAMA; 290[2]: 197). JAMA 2003; 289: 2560-2572.

[26] Chobanian AV, Bakris GL, Black HR, *et al.*: National Heart, Lung, and Blood Institute Joint National Committee on Prevention, Detection, Evaluation, and Treatment of High Blood pressure. National Heart, Lung, and Blood Institute; National High Blood Pressure Education Program Coordinating Committee. Seventh Report of the Joint National Committee on Prevention, Detection, Evaluation, and Treatment of High Blood Pressure. Hypertension 2003; 42: 1206-1252.

[27] American Heart Association. Understanding blood pressure readings 2010. Available at: http://www.americanheart.org/presenter.jhtml?identifier=2112.

[28] Effects of weight loss and sodium reduction intervention on blood pressure and hypertension incidence in overweight people with high-normal blood pressure. The Trials of Hypertension Prevention, phase II. The Trials of Hypertension Prevention Collaborative Research Group. Arch Intern Med 1997; 157: 657-667.

[29]   He J, Whelton PK, Appel LJ, Charleston J, Klag MJ. Long-term effects of weight loss and dietary sodium and the Dietary Approaches to Stop Hypertension (DASH) diet. DASH-Sodium Collaborative Research Group. N Eng J Med 2001; 344: 3-10.

[30]   Kelley GA. Kelley KS. Progressive resistance exercise and resting blood pressure: a meta-analysis of randomized controlled trials. Hypertension 2000; 35: 838-843.

[31]   Sacks FM, Svetkey LP, Vollmer WM, *et al*.: DASH-Sodium Collaborative Research Group. Effects on blood pressure of reduced dietary sodium and the Dietary Approaches to Stop Hypertension (DASH) diet. DASH-Sodium Collaborative Research Group. N Eng J MED 2001; 344: 3-10.

[32]   Vollmer WM, Sacks FM, Ard J, *et al*.: DASH-Sodium Collaborative Research Group. Effects of diet and sodium intake on blood pressure: subgroup analysis of the DASH-sodium trial. Ann Intern Med 2001; 135: 1019-1028.

[33]   Chobanian AV, Hill M. National Heart, Lung, and Blood Institute Workshop on Sodium and Blood pressure: a critical review of current scientific evidence. Hypertension 2000; 35: 858-863.

[34]   Neal B, MacMahon S, Chapman N. Blood Pressure Lowering Treatment Trialists' Collaboration. Lancet 2000; 356(9246): 1955-1964.

[35]   Franklin Roosevelt Presidential Library and Museum. Roosevelt Facts and Figures 2012. Available at: www.fdrlibrary.marist.edu/facts.html/

CHAPTER 12

The Othello Syndrome

Abstract: The dramatic works of William Shakespeare have left readers and audience members spellbound for centuries. Shakespeare explores many topics of the human experience in a manner which can, at times, be all too realistic as he starkly demonstrates the many aspects of the dark side of human nature. In the play, 'The Tragedy of Othello, the Moor of Venice', Shakespeare explores the effects of morbid jealousy.

The actions of the fictional character, Othello, has inspired modern psychological experts to refer to morbid jealousy as 'The Othello Syndrome'.

Keywords: Desdemona, economic stresses, extramarital sex, Iago, insecurity, morbid jealousy, murder, Othello Syndrome, Othello, playwright, psychiatric, Roderigo, sexual dysfunction, unfaithfulness.

WILLIAM SHAKESPEARE

William Shakespeare was an English playwright and poet. Shakespeare is considered, by literary experts, to be the greatest writer in the history of the English language. That is about all the experts can agree upon concerning the life and works of Shakespeare. Approximately 400 years after his death, Shakespeare is studied in every university throughout the world. Scholars devote their lives to studying and researching his works. His plays are revered and are performed on stage in all major cities at any given time. However, therein lies the rub.

Why don't we know more about the author of these works which have enchanted audiences and readers for centuries? Why are there no original manuscripts or notes of Shakespeare in existence? Perhaps the answer is that the actual individual named William Shakespeare might not have been the true author of any of the works attributed to Shakespeare. Many scholars today feel that this relatively uneducated, untravelled man would not be capable of writing the works of a genius which contain such intimate knowledge of the royal court, details of foreign cities, and the inner workings of various matters of commerce. Some candidates for the genuine author are Francis Bacon, Christopher Marlowe, and Edward de Vere, the 17th Earl of Oxford. My personal pick is William Strachey. Strachey was a passenger aboard the ship that is thought to have inspired 'The Tempest.'

What we do know of Shakespeare is that he was baptized at Holy Trinity Church in Stratford-Upon-Avon on April 26, 1564. From this baptismal date scholars assume that April 23, 1564 is Shakespeare's real birthday because no birth records exist.

On November 28, 1582 Shakespeare married Anne Hathaway. Hathaway was 8 years Shakespeare's senior and was pregnant at the time the two were married.

By the early 1590's Shakespeare had become involved in the theater and became a part-owner of The Globe Theater. Shakespeare's canonical work is considered to consist of 5 epic poems, 36 plays, and 154 sonnets.

Shakespeare died, according to legend on his birthday, April 23, 1616. However, this is probably merely a myth as Trinity Church records show that he was interred on April 5, 1616. The greatest playwright of all-time was survived by his wife, Anne, to whom he left, in his will, his 'second-best bed'.

WILLIAM SHAKESPEARE'S FICTIONAL CHARACTER OTHELLO

Othello is the title character in Shakespeare's play- The Tragedy of Othello, the Moor of Venice. Othello is a Moorish general in the Venetian army. The play opens with another character, Roderigo, learning that Othello has married the woman, Desdemona, that he had desired to be his own wife. Roderigo tells his feelings to Iago. Iago, in turn tells Roderigo of his hatred for Othello because he had promoted another soldier, Michael Cassio, instead of himself.

Iago informs Desdemona's father who later accuses Othello of seducing his daughter by witchcraft. Othello denies this vehemently and Desdemona supports him by stating that she married him because of true love.

The Duke of Venice appoints Othello as General of the Defense against the Turks. Desdemona receives permission to follow Othello to Cyprus. She is placed in a ship with the treacherous Iago and his wife, Emilia.

While in Cyprus, Iago places doubts in the mind of Othello concerning the love and faithfulness of Desdemona. He states that she is truly in love with Cassio. Cassio is subsequently demoted.

Iago arranges a meeting between Cassio and Desdemona. Cassio asks Desdemona to speak on his behalf to her husband to regain his old position. Both during and after the meeting Iago continues to cast doubts into the mind of Othello. Othello asks Iago to prove that Desdemona is unfaithful. Iago continues to provide whatever proof which might convince Othello of his wife's unfaithfulness.

Othello is now thoroughly convinced of his wife's unfaithfulness and plots to kill her.

Iago promises to kill Cassio. Othello confronts his wife and accuses her of being unfaithful. Desdemona is shocked and professes her love for Othello.

Roderigo and Iago attack Cassio. Moments later Othello murders the innocent Desdemona by smothering her with a pillow. Soon thereafter Othello is informed of Iago's ruse. Othello stabs himself and dies on the bed next to Desdemona.

THE OTHELLO SYNDROME

Othello erroneously thought there was a romantic relationship between his wife, Desdemona, and Cassio. Although there was no such relationship between the two and the jealousy did not have any factual roots, the jealousy that raged from the soul of Othello was real. This form of jealousy would be categorized today as morbid jealousy. Psychiatrists have coined the term 'Othello Syndrome' to describe this particular form of jealousy.

Morbid jealousy is defined as being a range of irrational thoughts and emotions, together with associated unacceptable behavior, in which the dominant theme is a preoccupation with a partner's sexual unfaithfulness based on unfounded evidence

[1]. This type of jealousy is not normal. Individuals, such as Othello, who are morbidly jealous take irrelevant occurrences as sound proof of their loved one's infidelity [2, 3].

It is thought by psychiatrists that there are four features of morbid jealousy [3, 4] which are the following: 1) an underlying mental disorder emerges before or with the jealousy; 2) the features of the underlying disorder coexist with the jealousy; 3) the course of morbid jealousy closely relates to that of the underlying disorder; 4) the jealousy has no basis in reality.

There are many causes of morbid jealousy. Research has shown that 15% of individuals with morbid jealousy possess an organic psychosyndrome with which the morbid jealousy is associated [5] while others have suffered some form of cerebral injury [1]. Still others [6] have suggested that feelings of insecurity, oversensitivity, and inadequacy are major predisposing factors of morbid jealousy and, in turn, individuals [7] with these characteristics are more likely to make systematic distortions and errors in their perceptions of events and various data which cause a precipitating event to give rise to incorrect assumptions and conclusions thus provoking morbid jealousy [3].

Researchers have documented the prevalence of morbid jealousy in men who, as adolescents, had seen their mothers engaged in extramarital sexual activity [8]. Other causes often cited as giving rise to morbid jealousy are various forms of sexual dysfunction [2, 9] and economic stresses [10].

REFERENCES

[1]   Cobb J. Morbid jealousy. British Journal of Hospital Medicine 1979; 21: 511-518.
[2]   Vauhkonen K. On the pathogenesis of morbid jealousy. Acta Psychiatrica Scandinavica Supplementum 1968; 202; 2-261.
[3]   Kingham M, Gordon H. Aspects of morbid jealousy. APT May 2004; 10: 207-215.
[4]   Mullen PE. Morbid jealousy and the delusion of infidelity. In Principles and Practice of Forensic Psychiatry (eds R. Bluglass & P. Bowden), pp. 823-834. London: Churchill Livingstone.
[5]   Mullen PE, Maack LH. Jealousy, pathological jealousy and aggression. In Aggression and Dangerousnes (Eds. D. P. Farrington & J. Gunn), 1985; pp. 103-126. London: Wiley.
[6]   Enoch MD, Trethowan WH. Uncommon Psychiatric Syndromes (2nd edn), 1979; pp. 25-40. Bristol: John Wright.

[7]   Tarrier N, Beckett R, Harwood S, *et al.* Morbid jealousy: a review and cognitive-behavioural formulation. Br J Psychiatry 1990; 157: 319-326.

[8]   Docherty JP, Ellis J. A New concept and finding in morbid jealousy. Am J Psychiatry 1976; 133: 679-683.

[9]   Todd J, Mackie JRM, Dewhurst K. Real or imagined hypophallism: a cause of inferiority feelings and morbid sexual jealousy. Br J Psychiatry 1971; 119: 315-318.

[10]   Shepherd M. Morbid jealousy: some clinical and social aspects of a psychiatric symptom. J Mental Sci 1961; 107: 688-704.

CHAPTER 13

The 1981 Irish Hunger Strikers

Abstract: In 1981 ten martyrs for the Irish Republican cause sacrificed themselves by participating in a hunger strike at Her Majesty's Prison Maze better known as The Maze, Long Kesh, or, simply, H Blocks in County Down, Ireland. The 1981 Hunger Strike was a direct confrontation between the Irish political prisoners and the Prime Minister of Great Britain, Margaret Thatcher. The 1981 Hunger Strike began on March 1 when The Irish Republican Army's Bobby Sands refused food. He would be joined by other brave men at staggered intervals. The Strike was called off when it became apparent that the families of these men would permit medical intervention, against the will of the strikers, when they would eventually slip into unconsciousness.

Keywords: 1981 Hunger Strike, Irish National Liberation Army, Irish Republican Army, starvation.

BOBBY SANDS

Bobby Sands was born in Belfast, Northern Ireland on March 9, 1954. Sands wrote of his childhood during which his family had to repeatedly move in order to avoid intimidation by British loyalists, "I was only a working-class boy from a Nationalist ghetto ... but it is repression that creates the revolutionary spirit of freedom" [1]. At the age of 18 he was forced out of his job as an apprentice car builder by a group of British supporters [1].

Soon thereafter, he found himself imprisoned at the Maze Prison. He was released from prison in 1976 and lived in relative freedom for a year before he was arrested again on handgun possession charges and sentenced to 14 years. This time he was sent to H-blocks where the British government had withdrawn 'special category status' in an attempt to criminalize the prisoners and delegitimatize the cause of Irish freedom and civil rights. He joined other prisoners in what was known as the 'blanket protest'. Subsequently, he was beaten regularly, placed in solitary confinement and given only bread and water to eat. Upon visiting the H-blocks, Catholic Archbishop Cardinal Tomas O Flaich compared the conditions to "the sewer pipes in the slums of Calcutta" [2].

On March 1, 1981 Sands became the first prisoner to refuse food thus beginning the Hunger Strike. His strike lasted for 66 days. He lapsed into a coma 48 hours prior to being declared dead by the medical staff at the Maze prison. He had lost 60 pounds during the nine week period.

News of Sands' death spread quickly throughout the world. Nelson Mandela was said to have been deeply influenced by Bobby Sands and later undertook his own hunger strike on Robben Island. In New York, the International Longshoremen's Association announced a 24-hour boycott of British ships.

Sands wrote, "Our revenge will be the laughter of our children". On the 20th anniversary of his martyrdom a commemorative mass was held for Sands in St. Patrick's Cathedral in New York City. His family was in attendance [3].

STARVATION

An average 70 kg man has fuel reserves of approximately 161,000 kcal. A typical daily energy need of such an individual is between 1,600 kcal and 6,000 kcal depending on one's activity level. Therefore, in times of starvation such an individual has stored fuels for 1 to 3 months.

The body undergoes various changes during starvation in order to attempt to compensate for the absence of caloric intake. Ketone bodies are considered to be equivalents of fatty acids. They are capable of passing through the blood-brain barrier. After several weeks of starvation fatty acids are effectively converted into ketone bodies by the liver and are used by the brain thus markedly diminishing the need for glucose [4].

Glycogen stores decrease rapidly in those individuals undergoing starvation. They also have a diminished ability to oxidize carbohydrates. In the final phase of starvation, before death, there is a critical exhaustion of body fat to a point where endogenous protein is needed for fuel [5].

THE ULTIMATE SACRIFICE

On March 1, 1981 Bobby Sands, leader of the Irish Republican Army (IRA) in the Maze Prison refused food thus commencing the Hunger Strike which would be transformative in the political landscape of Northern Ireland. The original aim of the strike could be considered to be small or almost insignificant to the outside observer. Ten Republican prisoners would starve themselves to death over the next seven months in support of their demands. The world would look on in shocked horror as one after another young man died a gruesome and self-inflicted martyr's death.

The concept of the hunger strike as a political tactic has deep roots within the Republican community. Terence MacSwiney was Lord Mayor of Cork. At MacSwiney's inauguration as Lord Mayor he stated, "It is not those who can inflict the most, but those who can suffer the most who will conquer". MacSwiney later died, in 1920, at Brixton Prison in London after being on a hunger strike for 74 days. His quote was often recalled during the 1981 Hunger Strike [6].

One tactic of the 1981 Hunger Strike which differed from previous hunger strikes is that the individual hunger strikers started to refuse food at different time intervals. This staggering tactic had the effect of producing single deaths on multiple days rather than a few deaths on a single day. This caused more media attention and heightened the drama as seen on the world's stage. It maximized the pressure being placed on the British government.

On March 15 Francis Hughes joined the strike. Raymond McCreesh of South Armagh and Patsy O'Hara of Derry City soon joined their fellow volunteers. All these men were in their twenties.

During the beginning phases of the strike Frank Maguire, Independent Nationalist member of Parliament, died. A special election was called for to elect a new member of Parliament to represent the people of Fermanagh/South Tyrone. On April 9, 1981, 30,492 people of Fermanagh/South Tyrone showed up at the polls to cast their vote for the imprisoned Bobby Sands then in his sixth week without food. Bobby Sands won the election and was now a member of the British

Parliament. It was thought that there was no possible way that the British Prime Minister, Margaret Thatcher, would stand by and allow a member of parliament die by starvation [7]. This notion proved to be incorrect.

66 days after the Hunger Strike began Bobby Sands became the first to sacrifice his life for the Republican cause. The British government remained unmoved publicly by the deaths of three more young men within the next two weeks.

Rev. Denis Faul, a Roman Catholic chaplain at Maze Prison, became a leader in the campaign to end the Hunger Strike. He stated, "Why should anybody's son be the last man to die?" The British government was starting to make some concessions by the end of July. However, they would make no concessions on freedom of association [8]. Two more martyrs, Joe McDonnell and Martin Hurson, had passed away by this point. On July 31 Paddy Quinn was the first to be taken off the strike as he was removed from it by his mother after having refused food for 47 days. This was followed by the deaths of Kevin Lynch, Kieran Doherty, Thomas McElwee and Michael Devine.

On the day that Michael Devine died, August 20, the wife of Pat McGeown interceded and asked for medical attention to spare her husband's life. As the hunger strikers would slip into unconsciousness other families would ask for medical intervention to save their loved one's life.

The Hunger Strike was reluctantly called off on October 3, 1981. Gerry Adams, future President of the Sinn Fein political party stated that "while we must adopt a compassionate and fraternal attitude to those families that intervened, one cannot underestimate the enormity of their action or the manner in which the defeatist and demoralizing campaign by some clergymen influenced their decision."

British Prime Minister Margaret Thatcher was awakened in Australia while attending the Commonwealth Conference with the welcome news that the Hunger Strike had been called off. She publicly refused to the end to grant the prisoners the political status which they desired [9]. The Hunger Strike brought worldwide attention and sympathy to the Republican cause. The result was huge amounts of monetary donations particularly from the United States.

In 1985 surviving hunger striker, Pat McGeown described the conditions inside the Maze prior to the strike, "There were times you would vomit. There were times when you were so run down that you would lie for days and not do anything with the maggots crawling all over you. The rain would be coming in the window and you would be lying there with the maggots all over the place" [10].

While Margaret Thatcher possessed a firm and unsympathetic public stance towards the desires of the strikers, such was not the case behind closed doors. Recently, released letters and files indicate that she was communicating with the prisoners through MI6, the British Secret Intelligence Service.

Thatcher stated to her cabinet that "further thought would need to be given to all possible courses of action in regard to Northern Ireland, however difficult or unpalatable" [9].

On July 6, 1981 a message was sent *via* MI6 to the leadership of the Provisional IRA through a Derry businessman, Brendan Duddy, who acted as an intermediary. The letter was an attempt to break a deal stating that the prisoners would be able to wear their own clothes. The letter was annotated in what appears to be the distinctive handwriting of Thatcher herself. The letter ends, "If the reply we receive is unsatisfactory and there is subsequently any public reference to this exchange we shall deny it took place. Silence will be taken as an unsatisfactory reply" [9].

One can only speculate as to how significant were the concessions which the so-called 'Iron Lady' was considering as she described them as being "difficult or unpalatable".

In September of 1997 United States Senator George Mitchell negotiated an agreement known as 'The Mitchell Principles of Democracy and Nonviolence'. It was agreed upon by the British government and Sinn Fein. It had six ground rules [11] to which all involved pledged "their commitment: to democratic and exclusively peaceful means of resolving political issues; to the total disarmament of all paramilitary organizations; to agree that such disarmament must be verifiable to the satisfaction of an independent commission; to renounce for themselves, and to oppose any effort by others, to use force, or threaten to use force, to influence the course or the outcome of all-party negotiations; to agree to abide by the terms of any agreement reached in all-party negotiations and to resort to democratic and exclusively peaceful methods in trying to alter any aspect of that outcome with which they may disagree; to urge that punishment killings and beatings stop and to take effective steps to prevent such actions [12, 13]."

REFERENCES

[1]   Bio.TrueStory. Bobby Sands. Accessed on August 11, 2013. Available at: http://www.biography.com/people/bobby-sands-26941955.
[2]   Bowcott O. The Guardian. Thatcher Cabinet 'Wobbled' over IRA Hunger Strikers. 12/29/11.
[3]   McShane L. The New York daily News. May 5, 2012. Death of bobby Sands in 1981 put human face to Northern Ireland's 'Troubles'.
[4]   Berg JM, Tymoczko JL,Stryer L. Biochemistry. 5th edition. New York: WH Freeman; 2002.
[5]   Comparative Physiology of Fasting, Starvation, and Food limitation (Ed.) M.D. McCue. 2012, XIII, 430p. 84 illus., 24 illus. in color, hardcover.
[6]   Cain. The Hunger Strike of 1981- Summary. Accessed on September 1, 2013. Available at: http://cain.ulst.ac.uk/events/hstrike/summary.htm
[7]   Irish Hunger Strike. The Ultimate Sacrifice. Accessed on August 18, 2013. Available at: http://www.irishhungerstrike.com/fasttildeath.htm
[8]   BBC. Republican Hunger Strikes. Accessed on August 26, 2013. Available at: http://www.bbc.co.uk/history/events/republican_hunger_strikes_maze
[9]   New York Times. October 4, 1981.
[10]   Bishop P, Mallie E.The provisional IRA. Corgi Books. 1981; p. 352.
[11]   Benton J. The Evolution of peace: the role of George Mitchell in the Northern Ireland peace process. Accessed on March 10, 2014. Available at: http://www.cumberlands.edu/academics/history/files/vol14/jbenton01.html.
[12]   Knox C, *et al*. Peacebuilding in Northern Ireland, Israel, and South Africa St. Martin's Press, LLC: 2000. page 39.
[13]   Studies in Conflict & Terrorism, Volume 25, Issue 1, 2002.

CHAPTER 14

Samuel Clemens Visits the Dentist

Abstract: American humorist and author Samuel Clemens was afflicted with periodontal disease. While living in Hartford, Connecticut his dentist was Dr. John Riggs who is considered to be the father of periodontics. Dr. Riggs studied under another Hartford dentist, Dr. Horace Wells. Dr. Wells is a pioneer in the field of anesthesia. In one of Clemens' posthumously published short stories, 'Happy Memories of the Dental Chair', Clemens gives insights into the origins of periodontics and anesthesia.

Keywords: Anesthesia, Elmira, hypersensitivity, nitrous oxide, oral hygiene, periodontics, periodontist.

SAMUEL CLEMENS

On November 30, 1835 Samuel Langhorne Clemens was born in the small town of Florida, Missouri. He had many vocations in his life- a riverboat pilot, journalist, inventor, soldier, miner and publisher. He became the most famous American humorist of all time and a prolific author. Ernest Hemingway described Clemens' magnum opus of 1884, 'The Adventures of Huckleberry Finn', as the work from which all other American literature emanated. When young Sam was four-years-old the family moved to a small town of 1,000 people. The town was Hannibal, Missouri and later became the beloved and almost magical setting of Clemens' tales of boyhood adventure.

Clemens' particular form of wit was a marriage between carefree musings and dark observational insights into everyday American life. This was probably the result of the polar personalities of his parents. Clemens' father, John, had a difficult life struggling to care for his family. It is said that Clemens never saw his own father laugh. On the other hand, Clemens' mother was a gregarious, warm homemaker who loved to tell her enchanted family nightly stories [1]. The personalities of his parents manifested themselves in Clemens' own tales of boyhood days in the river towns. On one hand they were sunlit, joyous days that were filled with boundless energy and unlimited potential for a bright future. On the other hand the days of his youthful characters were filled with boredom, stress, death, prejudice, and poverty. This dichotomy was a microcosm of Clemens' own youth. Evidently, Clemens believed in his own quote, "write what you know".

When Clemens was 12-years-old his father died. This marked the end of his formal education. Sam was apprenticed to a printer named Ament who paid him in board and clothes. Clemens later described his wages as being "more board than clothes". Clemens subsequently left Ament and started working for his brother, Orion. The two brothers run a small Hannibal newspaper. When Orion was away, Sam would write and publish his own articles. These articles would usually be a commentary or satire of local characters or conditions. These satirical musings of the youngster were written in a manner which became familiar to readers worldwide decades later. Obviously, these articles caused untold grief and problems for older brother Orion upon his return to the newspaper office. However, the articles sold papers and they made a profit [2] which was very unusual in the newspaper business at that time. Clemens would move about the country working in various positions in printing and publishing. He eventually went to New Orleans, Louisiana where he became one of the most trusted and respected pilots of the Mississippi River. This entailed an acquisition of an incredible amount of knowledge concerning every detail of the twelve hundred mile river.

In 1861 Clemens took a steamer north. Upon reaching St. Louis, Missouri a blank cartridge was fired at the ship from Jefferson Barracks. The message the artillerymen were trying to give to the ship was not understood and it proceeded traveling north. Subsequently, a shell carried away part of the pilot-house. It was not until then that Clemens and his fellow occupants of the pilot-house realized that the American Civil War had begun.

Clemens hurried back to Hannibal and joined the military. Clemens once said "war was invented so Americans could learn geography". After a military career of two rainy weeks Clemens decided it was an appropriate time to start learning geography in a somewhat safer and comfortable manner. He resigned from the military and set out for Nevada with Orion who had been appointed Secretary of the new territory.

While out west, Clemens occasionally wrote small articles, under the pen name of Josh, for the Virginia City Enterprise in an effort to survive financially. He was eventually offered the position of local editor. At this point he changed his pen name to Mark Twain, a river term which brought back precious memories of his days on the Mississippi River. Twain subsequently wrote for many other newspapers while continuing to keep involved in many varied professions.

Clemens headed for Calaveras County to mine gold and found this work very disagreeable. He and his friend, Jim Gillis, filed a claim-notice for an area in which they had found a little gold. It started to rain and Clemens had no part of the inclement weather so he returned to camp for the next three weeks never to visit again the area they had claimed.

They let the claim-notice expire. The rain exposed solid gold nuggets which were previously covered by only a thin layer of soil. While others were staking out Clemens' rightful gold fortune he was spending his time writing a story about a frog. To be specific- a frog that had great jumping talents. This story was first published in The Saturday Press on November 18, 1865 as 'Jim Smiley and His Jumping Frog' later to be published as 'The Celebrated Jumping Frog of Calaveras County'. This became Clemens' first popular success. It was rapidly translated into many languages and bringing Clemens worldwide fame. His life never remained the same. Clemens spent the next few years giving lectures and writing many travel essays. In Elmira, New York he met Olivia Langdon. She was 22-years-old and became Clemens' editor- a position she would hold for the rest of her life. On February 2, 1870 Clemens and Olivia got married. The couple moved to Hartford, Connecticut and it was there that their first-born child, Langdon, died in 1872. It was in the Hartford house, along with summer trips to Elmira, that Clemens authored some of the most notable works in American literature.

Financial disaster haunted Clemens despite his many best-selling works. In 1895 he set about a triumphant world tour to repay his debts and rebuild the family fortune. However, misfortune again walked hand-in-hand with Clemens' joys. A message reached Clemens in England that his daughter, Susy, had died. He could not even make it home in time for her burial. In 1903, Mrs. Clemens died in Florence, Italy and was brought home to Elmira to be buried next to Susy.

Clemens returned to America saying, "Travel has no longer any charm for me. I have seen all the foreign countries I want to except heaven and hell and I only have a vague curiosity about one of them." However, he gladly set sail for England in 1907 when the University of Oxford granted him an honorary degree. Clemens was very aware that one of the greatest universities in the world honoring the former poverty-stricken boy from the riverbanks of the Mississippi was to be the pinnacle of his career.

On Christmas Eve 1909 Clemens' daughter, Jean, died of an epileptic seizure. This prompted Clemens to state, "I never greatly envied anybody but the dead". Clemens followed Jean into the eternal peace he so desired only a few months later. He was buried in Elmira, New York and his grave is marked by a headstone which is twelve feet tall- two fathoms or, in Mississippi River pilot terminology, a 'mark twain'.

DR. JOHN MANKEY RIGGS

Dr. John M. Riggs was born in Seymour, Connecticut on October 25, 1811. Dr. Riggs was the first person to limit his dental practice to periodontics and is considered to be the first periodontist [3]. He is also known as 'the father of the therapeutic approach' to treating periodontal disease [4]. Riggs was very progressive in his approach to periodontal treatment. He stressed the importance of oral hygiene and prevention [5, 6]. This approach was presented to The International Medical Congress in 1881. Periodontal disease was, at one time, referred to as Riggs' Disease.

DR. HORACE WELLS

Horace Wells was a practicing dentist in Hartford, Connecticut during the 1840's. Wells, on the morning of December 10, 1844, noticed an advertisement in The Hartford Courant for a demonstration- "A Grand Exhibition of the Effects

Produced by Inhaling Nitrous Oxide, Exhilarating, or Laughing Gas" [7]. Wells decided to attend this demonstration, with his wife, put on by Gardner Quincy Colton [8]. Wells had the vision to see that this gas might be able to provide surgical patients with the much sought after relief from pain that the medical community desired to provide.

After several successful employments of nitrous oxide as an anesthesia, Wells demonstrated its use at Massachusetts General Hospital. The demonstration was considered a fiasco, at the time, and Wells returned to Hartford a shell of his former self. Wells and his reputation never recovered from this failed demonstration [4].

William Morton, two years later, gave a definitive demonstration of inhalation ether. Morton was a former student of Wells [9]. Morton received much of the praise for his work in developing anesthesia. Wells did not, in his day, receive the credit he deserved for being a pioneer in anesthesia research even though he truly made great contributions to the burgeoning field of medical anesthesiology.

Wells was arrested in New York City in 1848 on his 33rd birthday. Wells subsequently committed suicide while in prison. Ironically, he anesthetized himself with chloroform prior to slashing his left femoral artery [9].

PERIODONTAL DISEASE

Periodontal disease refers to a disease process which can range from inflammation of the gingiva to destruction of the soft tissue and bone which provide support to the teeth. There are certain known risk factors for periodontal disease. These include smoking, hormonal changes in females, diabetes, medications, and various illnesses [10].

There can be warning signs of periodontal disease. Such warning signs can include bad breath or bad taste which does not disappear, red or swollen gingiva, painful chewing, loose teeth, sensitive teeth, gingival recession, change in occlusion of teeth, and a change in fit of existing removable partial dentures [11].

Periodontal disease can affect up to 90% of the worldwide population [12]. There is an immune-inflammatory response which develops in the periodontal tissues in response to the chronic presence of plaque bacteria. This response results in the destruction of the periodontium's structural components [13]. Presently, for non-surgical management of chronic periodontitis, scaling and root planing are the accepted treatment modality [14]. The prevention of periodontal disease starts with education.

Individuals need to see their dentist on a regular basis and receive proper periodontal treatment. The treatment of periodontal disease does not start and end in the dentist's office. Rather, it is imperative that individuals perform proper oral home care as directed and instructed by their dentist. This includes proper brushing and flossing techniques. Re-evaluation visits scheduled at proper intervals are an imperative part of proper periodontal therapy.

MARK TWAIN GOES TO THE PERIODONTIST

In April of 2009, a short story, authored by Clemens, was published. It was entitled 'Happy Memories of the Dental Chair' [15] and was written over a hundred years prior to its publication. It was originally intended to be published during Clemens' life but he decided against its publication mainly because of the manner by which he describes his dentist and personal friend, Dr. John Riggs. He describes Riggs as having "the calm, possessed, surgical look of a man who could endure pain in another person". Riggs himself surely would have not been offended by this description of himself penned by his acerbically witty friend. However, Riggs died shortly after the story was written and Clemens didn't want Riggs' family to read such a description of a truly distinguished gentleman.

In this short story Clemens, in his unique manner, gives the reader a glimpse into the 19th century dental practice. This is particularly important for two reasons. The first is Clemens relates what Dr. Riggs told him of the birth of anesthesia and the beliefs and theories of Dr. Riggs concerning periodontal therapy.

The reader is told of the evening in December of 1844 when Dr. Wells attended Gardiner Colton's nitrous oxide exhibition. Clemens relates how Wells was struck with the wondrous possibilities of using nitrous oxide to alleviate pain during surgery.

At the time, Dr. Riggs was a student of Dr. Wells. Wells asked Colton to come to his office the next morning with the nitrous oxide. Riggs goes on to tell Clemens of how he extracted one of Wells' third molars that morning utilizing nitrous oxide anesthesia. Clemens proceeds to tell the reader that he was initially referred to Dr. Riggs by another dentist because of the severity of his periodontal condition and Dr. Riggs' success in treating such conditions. He states that Riggs has a method of treating the disease which "in some instances arrested its progress and rendered it harmless in all" [15]. Riggs proceeds to examine Clemens and describes the course of treatment. Riggs starts the periodontal treatment as he 'put(s) his tool into my mouth, rooted it up under a gum and began to carve' [15]. Clemens further describes the sensitivity to cold which followed the periodontal treatment in what could be described as the first-ever written account of post-operative hypersensitivity. Clemens even comments on the importance of oral hygiene and prevention which were hallmarks of Dr. Riggs throughout his career [3].

REFERENCES

[1]   Bio.True Story. Mark Twain Biography. Accessed on October 1, 2012. Available at: http://www.biography.com/people/mark-twain-9512564.
[2]   The Complete Works of Mark Twain. Mark Twain Biography. Accessed on August 31, 2012. Available at: http://www.mtwain.com.
[3]   Shklar G. Carranza FA. The historical background of periodontology. In: Carranza's clinical periodontolgy. 9th ed. Newman MG, Takei HH, Carranza FA, editors. Philadelphia: W.B. Saunders Company. p. 7.
[4]   Maloney WJ. A Periodontal case report by Dr. S.L. Clemens. J Dent Res 2010; 89(7): 676-678.
[5]   Riggs JM. Suppurative inflammation of the gums and absorption of the gums and alveolar process. Penn J Dent Sci 3: 99. Reprinted in Arch Clin Oral Pathol (1938) 2: 423.
[6]   MacManus C. The makers of dentistry. Dent Cosmos 1902; 44: 1105.
[7]   Hartford Courant. December 10, 1844.
[8]   Wildsmith JA, Menczer LF. A British footnote to the life of Horace Wells. Br J Anesth 59: 1067-1069.
[9]   Finder SG. Lessons from history: Horace Wells and the moral features of clinical contexts. Anesth Prog 42: 1-6.
[10]   National Institute of Dental and Craniofacial Research. Periodontal (Gum) Disease: Causes, Symptoms, and Treatments. Accessed on December 25, 2012. Available at: http://www.

nidcr.nih.gov/nidcrZ.nih.gov/Templates/CommonPage.aspx?NRMODE=Published&NRN
ODEGUID=%7bcEZ46689-D899-4cc7-B68A-805AD10F4E7%67d&NRORIGINALURL
=%2fOralHealth%2fTopics%62fGumDiseases%2fPeriodontalGumDisease%2ehtm&NRC
ACHEHINT=Guest#intro.

[11]   Centers for Disease Control and Prevention. Warning signs. Accessed on January 1, 2013. Available at: http://www.cdc.gov/oralhealth/topics/periodontal_disease.htm.

[12]   Philstrom BL, Michalowicz BS, Johnson NW. Periodontal diseases. Lancet 2005 Nov 19; 366(9499): 1809-1820.

[13]   Preshaw PM, Seymour RA, Heasman PA. Current concepts in periodontal pathogenesis. Dent Update 2004 Dec; 31(10): 570-572, 574-578.

[14]   Cobb CM. Microbes, inflammation, scaling and root planing, and the periodontal condition. J Dent Hyg 2008 Oct; 82 Suppl 3: 4-9.

[15]   Twain M. Happy memories of the dental chair. In: Who is Mark Twain? Hirst RH, editor, New York, NY: Harper Collins, pp. 77-85.

CHAPTER 15

The Bell's Palsy of Lisa Gherardini: The Solution to the Enigma of the Mona Lisa's Smile

Abstract: The smile of 'The Mona Lisa' has enchanted researchers, art enthusiasts, and historians for centuries. The smile can best be described as being enigmatic. Academicians have presented numerous theories in an attempt to explain the nature of the smile through the use of both modern technology and various documented facts concerning the portrait. The true origin of the smile can finally be revealed. I theorize that the smile is the direct result of the masterful representation of a woman who had recently given birth and was affected by Bell's palsy. Bell's palsy is a condition which is more commonly found in individuals who are either pregnant or have recently given birth.

Keywords: Art, Bell's palsy, decreased tearing, dizziness, electromyography, facial nerve, gestational hypertension, Giocondo, hyperacusis, impaired taste, Mona Lisa, preeclampsia, pregnancy, puerperium, smile, viral infection.

LEONARDO DA VINCI

On April 15, 1452, in the town of Vinci, Italy, one of the greatest minds in the history of mankind was born. Leonardo was born, like so many others who would eventually obtain greatness in their lifetimes, into the most humble of origins. Leonardo was the illegitimate son of a 25-year old notary and a peasant girl. Leonardo had seventeen half siblings.

Leonardo's father brought some examples of the child's art to a friend who was an artist, Andrea del Verrocchio [1]. The artist was astounded by the youth's talent. He allowed Leonardo to start studying in his workshop. Leonardo studied many branches of art such as sculpture, drawing, and painting. Leonardo became very proficient in architecture and geometry. However, a trait became apparent which would follow Leonardo, as well as many geniuses, for the rest of his life. Leonardo had difficulty finishing tasks. He would lose interest and become very frustrated with small imperfections in his work. Young Leonardo could not accept the fact that his work was only that of a human. He always sought new challenges.

Leonardo's first major work was to paint an angel on Andrea's 'Baptism of Christ'. It was so superior to the master's own work that Andrea swore never to paint again after witnessing the youth's work.

In 1482, Leonardo entered into the service of Duke Ludovico Sforza. This relationship lasted 17 years and was a period of great scientific and artistic achievement for Leonardo. Between 1490 and 1495 Leonardo concentrated on four main themes- mechanics, human anatomy, architecture, and painting. Duke Ludovico Sforza fell from power in 1499 leaving Leonardo to search for a new patron. During the 17 years in service to the Duke, Leonardo only completed six works. However, of these six works two were 'The Last Supper' and 'The Virgin on the Rocks'.

Leonardo was in service to a few different patrons for the remaining years of his life. These patrons included Cesare Borgia, Niccolo Machiavelli, the Pope, and Giuliano de Medici. Leonardo passed away on May 2, 1519 in Cloux, France. The man that some had, years earlier, referred to as a commoner died in the arms of his final patron- Francis I, King of France.

LISA GHERARDINI AND 'THE MONA LISA'

On June 15, 1479 a baby girl was born in an old Florentine house. She was given the name Lisa. The house where she was born was previously used as a workshop by the local wool artisans. Sixteen years later Lisa married a local merchant, Francesco del Giocondo, who was twice her age. Francesco's previous wife had passed away approximately one year prior. The marriage of Francesco and Lisa produced five children- Piero, Andrea, Giocondo, Camilla, and Marietta.

Francesco del Giocondo, in 1503, commissioned Leonardo to produce a portrait of his beautiful wife, Lisa. The reason Francesco sought to have this portrait produced is integral in solving the enigma of the smile of 'The Mona Lisa". Presently, the portrait resides in the Louvre in France. The Louvre offers a few possible theories as to the reason the portrait was commissioned. My personal belief is that it was to celebrate the birth of the couple's second son, Andrea, who was born in December of 1502.

For the past five centuries people have debated about the identity of the model for 'The Mona Lisa'. In 2008, a group of German academics headed by Dr. Armin Schlechter solved the mystery. They discovered notes scribbled in the margins of a book in October of 1503 which confirmed that Lisa Gherardini was the model for the famed portrait.

In 2004, the French Museum's Center for Research and Restoration used laser scanning on the portrait. It showed the model to be wearing a very fine gauze veil on her dress. This was indicative of a woman who was either pregnant or who had very recently given birth. Laser and infrared scans were used by the National Research Council of Canada to show that the model's hair was originally in a bun. This detail was hidden by varnish and darkened paint. It was common practice in the 16th century for Italian women who were either pregnant or had recently given birth to place their hair in a bun.

Adour [2] deserves credit for introducing "the theory that the enigmatic smile of" 'The Mona Lisa' "was an artistic representation of the facial" musculature "contracture that develops subsequent to" Bell's "palsy when the facial nerve has undergone partial Wallerian degeneration and has" regenerated. The medical community has elaborated on this topic over the past two decades [3].

Lisa Gherardini passed away at the age of 63. She was buried at the Convent of Sant'Orsola where her youngest child, Marietta, lived as a nun. There have been a few recent attempts to find Lisa's body at this convent. These attempts have proven, so far, to be fruitless.

BELL'S PALSY

Bell's palsy is a form of a temporary facial paralysis. It is caused by one of the two facial nerves being damaged. It can affect all ages and both sexes. There are various theories concerning the etiology [4-6] of Bell's palsy. Possible cause are viral infection, vascular ischemia, autoimmune disorders [6, 9, 10], and the reactivation of herpes simplex virus in the geniculate ganglia [7, 8].

Facial expressions such as smiling, frowning, and blinking are controlled by the facial nerve. Bell's palsy can cause impaired taste hyperacusis, pain around the ar, decreased tearing [6, 10], impaired speech, difficulty eating and drinking, and dizziness. The cause of Bell's palsy is one of the two facial nerves being damaged. It occurs at a rate of 45.1/100,000 in pregnant women [11, 12] which is much higher than in the non-pregnant population. Most of these cases occur either in the third trimester or immediately after giving birth [12, 13]. It is thought to be caused by the increased extracellular volume in mothers or certain nerve compression syndromes which occur in the final stages of pregnancy [12, 14, 15]. There also seems to be a correlation between Bell's palsy and preeclampsia [16, 17].

REFERENCES

[1]   Vasari G (1896). Life of Leonardo da Vinci. In: Lives of the most eminent painters, sculptors, and architects. 1896; Translated De Vere G du C. London: Scribner's, pp. 89-92, 95-101, 104-105.

[2]   Adour KK. Mona Lisa syndrome: solving the enigma of the Gioconda smile. Ann Otol Rhinol Laryngol 1999. 98: 196-199.

[3]   Hellebrand MC, Friebe-Hoffmann U, Bender HG, Kojda G, Hoffmann TK. Das Mona-Lisa-Syndrom-die periphere Fazialisparese in der Schwangerschaft. Z Geburtshilfe Neonatol 2006. 210: 126-134.

[4]   Katusic SK, Beard CM, Wiederholt WC, Bergstralh EJ, Kurland LT (1986). Incidence, clinical features, and prognosis in Bell's palsy, Rochester, MN, 1968-1982. Ann Neurol 20: 622-627.

[5]   Peitersen E (2002). Bell's palsy, the spontaneous course of 2,500 peripheral facial nerve palsies of different etiologies. Acta Otolaryngol Suppl 549: 4-30.

[6]   Tsai HS, Chang LY, Lu CY, Lee PI, Chen JM, Lee CY, *et al.* (2009). Epidemiology and treatment of Bell's palsy in children in northern Taiwan. J Microbiol Immunol Infect 42: 351-356.

[7]   Murakami S, Mizobuchi M, Nakashiro Y, Doi T, Hato N, Yanagihara N. Bell palsy and herpes simplex virus: identification of viral DNA in endoneurial fluid and muscle. Ann Intern Med 1996; 124(1 Pt 1): 27-30.

[8]   Rowlands S, Hooper R, Hughes R, Burney P. The epidemiology and treatment of Bell's palsy in the UK. Eur J Neurol 9: 63-67.

[9]   Adour KK, Byl FM, Hilsinger RL Jr, Kahn ZM, Sheldon MI. The True nature of Bell's palsy: analysis of 1000 consecutive patients. Laryngoscope1978; 88: 787-801.

[10]   Singhi P, Jain V. Bell's palsy in children. Semin Pediatr Neurol 2003; 10: 289-297.

[11]   Hilsinger RL Jr, Adour KK, Doty HE. Idiopathic facial paralysis, pregnancy, and the menstrual cycle. Ann Otol Rhinol Laryngol 1975; 84(4 Pt 1): 433-442.

[12]   Shmorgun D, Chan WS, Ray JG. Association between Bell's palsy in pregnancy and pre-eclampsia. QJM 2002; 95: 359-362.

[13]   Shapiro JL, Yudin MH, Ray JG. Bell's palsy and tinnituis during pregnancy: predictors of pre-eclampsia. Acta Otolaryngol (Stockh)1999; 119: 647-651.

[14]   Davison JM. Edema in pregnancy. Kidney Int Suppl 1997; 59: 90-96.
[15]   Graham JG. Neurological complications of pregnancy and anesthesia. Clin Obstet Gynecol 1982; 9: 333-341.
[16]   Kovo M, Sagi Y, Lampl Y, Golan A. Simultaneous bilateral Bell's palsy during pregnancy. J Matern Fetal Neonatal Med 2009; 22: 1211-1213.
[17]   Mylonas I, Kastner R, Sattler C, Kainer F, Friese K. Idiopathic facial paralysis (Bell's palsy) in the immediate puerperium in a patient with mild preeclampsia: a case report. Arch Gynecol Obstet 2005; 272: 241-243.

CHAPTER 16

The Clandestine Oral Surgery of President Grover Cleveland

Abstract: Grover Cleveland was the first, and only, president of the United States to serve two non-consecutive terms. During Cleveland's second term the United States was experiencing a serious crisis which threatened the financial well-being of the nation. The magnitude of the crisis was not revealed to the public. Cleveland planned to ask Congress to repeal the Sherman Silver Purchase Act of 1890. He thought that a powerful speech before Congress could help avoid financial disaster. Shortly before scheduling his speech, a life-threatening growth was discovered in the President's mouth. A biopsy returned a diagnosis of cancer for the rough spot on the President's palate and surgical intervention would be required. A clandestine surgical team was assembled and successful surgeries were performed aboard a boat belonging to Cleveland's friend. Later, a prosthesis was constructed for the President to hide the physical effects of the surgery. Cleveland was able to make an eloquent speech before Congress, the Act was repealed and financial ruin for the nation was averted.

Keywords: Ackerman's tumor, alcohol, Buschke-Loewenstein tumor, cigarettes, florid oral papillomatosis, human papillomavirus, oral verrucous carcinoma, prosthodontics, Sherman Silver Purchase Act of 1890, tobacco, verrucous hyperplasia.

PRESIDENT GROVER CLEVELAND

On March 18, 1837 Reverend Richard Cleveland and his wife, Ann celebrated the birth of their son, Stephen Grover Cleveland. The couple named their son in honor of the first ordained pastor of the first Presbyterian Church in Caldwell, New Jersey [1].

Grover Cleveland was a very conservative individual in both a political and social manner. He is the only president of the United States to be elected to two non-consecutive terms. He is considered to be the twenty-second and twenty-fourth presidents of the United States [2].

President Cleveland is considered to be the last American president to largely ignore the press and trust his own instincts to guide him in setting public policies [3]. In foreign affairs, Cleveland most notably sent warships to South America to force mediation of a dispute between Venezuela and Great Britain in compliance with the principles of the Monroe Doctrine [4].

Later in life, Cleveland became closely associated with the life insurance business. He held the position of Chairman of the Executive Committee of the Association of Life Insurance Presidents and served as a rebate referee for the Mutual, Equitable, and New York Life Insurance Companies [5].

ORAL VERRUCOUS CARCINOMA

Oral verrucous carcinoma is a form of well differentiated squamous cell carcinoma [6]. In 1948, Lauren Ackerman [7] first described it as having both a distinctive morphological appearance and clinical behavior. Ackerman distinguished verrucous carcinoma from other epidermoid carcinomas based on its prognosis which is excellent when proper medical treatment is provided to the patient.

Oral verrucous carcinoma has been described in the scientific literature as epithelioma cuniculatum, Buschke-Loewenstein tumor, Ackerman's tumor, carcinoma cuniculatum, and florid oral papillomatosis [6, 8]. It has a predilection for the mucous membranes of the head and neck. It is found primarily in the oral cavity and, secondarily, in the larynx [9].

The etiology of verrucous carcinoma can best be described as being poorly defined [6]. Chewing tobacco [9] is a known etiologic factor in oral cavity lesions while cigarette smoking has a high correlation only with laryngeal lesions [6], the human papillomavirus [10], and the presence of oral lichenoid are all considered to be causative factors. An inflammatory involvement [11] can cause regional lymph nodes to become tender and enlarged.

Verrucous carcinoma is most prevalent in India [12] and occurs most often in elderly men. The high rate of verrucous carcinoma in India is probably due to the habitual chewing of pan [13]. The diagnosis of verrucous carcinoma [14] is based upon the extension of the lesion into the underlying connective tissue deep to the adjacent normal epithelium.

The available options for treatment have not been altered, to a great degree, since the days of Ackerman. Surgery or radiotherapy are the primary options to treat both the lesions of the oral cavity and the larynx. The surgical option has been demonstrated to be the more effective [9] of the two options. However, two studies [15, 16] have achieved comparably positive results using radiation to treat laryngeal verrucous carcinoma.

There has been much progress in developing more effective methods to close the oral defect created by the surgery since the days of Grover Cleveland. Aytekin *et al*. have had enormous success in reconstructing a defect in the oral cavity resulting from verrucous carcinoma. They employed a prefabricated parietal galeal flap [17].

The prognosis for treated verrucous carcinoma is excellent. Nevertheless, careful follow-up examinations are of paramount importance as verrucous carcinoma has the potential for local recurrence [18].

THE CLANDESTINE PRESIDENTIAL SURGERIES

An economic crisis threatened the financial well-being of the United States in 1883. Economists and politicians were torn on the issue of backing the United States currency by both gold and silver. The Sherman Silver Purchase Act of 1890 forced the United States Treasury to purchase large amounts of silver each month while allowing the redemption of United States Treasury notes in either gold or silver. A result of this Act was the rapid depletion of the Treasury's gold supply. President Cleveland thought that financial disaster could be averted by the repeal of the Act and he planned to make a speech before Congress on this account. The vice-president was Adlai Stevenson who was a strong silver advocate.

Cleveland noticed a rough patch on his palate in March of 1893. Dr. R.M. O'Reilly examined the area on June 18, 1893. It was noted to be about the size of a quarter dollar and it went from Cleveland's maxillary molars to within one-third of an inch of the midline. It encroached slightly onto the soft palate. Diseased bone was present and a specimen was sent to the pathologist at the Army Medical Museum. The pathologist did not know the identity of the patient and stated that there was probably a malignancy and surgical intervention would be needed.

The White House decided that the operation would have to be performed in absolute secrecy to prevent panic from spreading across America. A secret surgical team, sworn to secrecy, was assembled. This team was told that they would be performing the difficult surgery aboard the yacht, 'Oneida', belonging to President Cleveland's friend, Commodore Elias Benedict. The saloon of Benedict's yacht was made into an operating room [5]. The surgical team and President Cleveland boarded the yacht on the evening of June 30, 1893. The surgical team consisted of Dr. Joseph Bryant, a New York surgeon; Dr. William Keen, a professor at Jefferson College; Dr. John Erdmann; Dr. Edward Janeway, a New York internist; and Dr. Hasbrouck, a New York dentist [19].

The next morning the yacht set sail up the East River of Manhattan. The yacht was in full view of the staff at Bellevue Hospital. The surgical team members stayed in the cabin of the yacht so as to not arouse suspicion [19]. Dr. Hasbrouck, the dentist, started the surgery by extracting Cleveland's maxillary left first and second premolars using nitrous oxide. Dr. Bryant continued the surgery. He made incisions in the palate while Dr. Janeway monitored Cleveland's pulse and general condition [19]. Both topical and injected cocaine were administered and were supplemented with ether. Dr. Bryant then resected part of the left maxilla. He was assisted by Drs. Keen and Erdmann [12].

The surgeons removed the remaining portion of the left maxilla, exclusive of the medial wall and infraorbital plate [12]. They packed the surgical wound with iodoform gauze [19]. The whole procedure took under an hour and a half. An injection of one-sixth of a grain of morphine was given to Cleveland for pain control.

Cleveland was actually able to get out of bed late the next day, July 2. On July 5 the yacht arrived at the President's home, Gray Gables, in Buzzard's Bay, Massachusetts. It was noted that Cleveland walked from the launch to his house with little apparent effort [19].

Dr. Bryant, on July 17, performed a second surgery to remove a small residual lesion [4]. Drs. Janeway, Erdmann and Keen joined Dr. Bryant on this surgical team. This surgery was performed aboard the same yacht while Cleveland was at Gray Gables. The surgery was performed entirely intraorally in an effort to avoid a scar. Cleveland loved spending summers at Gray Gables which he did until 1904 when his 13 year-old daughter, Ruth, died of diphtheria [20].

A large defect was present in Cleveland's mouth as a result of the first surgery. A prosthesis made from vulcanized rubber was made by a New York prosthodontist, Dr. Kasson C. Gibson, for Cleveland. It supported the cheek and did not affect Cleveland's speech. A second prosthesis was made in October of 1893 by Dr. Gibson which the President truly treasured [21, 22].

It was not until the 20th century that President Cleveland's cancer was formally diagnosed. Modern equipment and techniques were employed to examine slides of the lesion. A diagnosis of oral verrucous carcinoma was obtained.

Also, many years later Dr. William Keen's recollections of Cleveland's surgeries were published in 'The Saturday Evening Post' on September 22, 1917. This was the first official acknowledgement that the surgeries ever took place. It was only published after Mrs. Thomas J. Preston, Jr., President Cleveland's widow, gave permission to finally divulge the secrets surrounding the surgeries. This permission was granted after a personal interview was conducted by Mrs. Preston.

AFTERMATH OF SURGERIES

The surgeries were a success but one can only speculate as to what would have been the economic fallout in the United States if the unthinkable had happened during these surgeries which were performed under such primitive conditions. Cleveland's surgeries clearly demonstrate the importance of oral cancer examinations and thorough head and neck examinations.

Today many dental professionals provide maxillofacial prostheses for individuals who have had head and neck cancer surgery. Similar to the wonderful work provided by President Cleveland's prosthodontist, Dr. Kasson C. Gibson, the maxillofacial prostheses restore form, function, and even some degree of happiness to cancer patients.

REFERENCES

[1]   New Jersey Division of Parks and Forestry. Grover Cleveland birthplace. accessed on March 17, 2014. Available at: www.state.nj.us/dep/parksandforests/historic/grover-cleveland/gc_earlyyears.htm.

[2]   Smithsonian Institution. Grover Cleveland 1837-1908. Accessed on March 17, 2014. Available at: americanhistory.si.edu/presidency/timeline/pres_era/3_683.html.

[3]   Graff HF. Grover Cleveland. Times Books; 2002; United States of America.

[4]   PBS. 22/24. Grover Cleveland. Accessed on March 17, 2014. Available at: www.pbs.org/wgbh/americanexperience/features/biography/presidents-cleveland/

[5]   The New York Times. Mr. Cleveland is dead. Page 1. June 25, 1908.

[6]   Alkan A, Bulot E, Gunhan O, Ozden B. Oral verrucous carcinoma: a study of 12 cases. Eur J Dent 2010 April; 4(2): 202-207.

[7]   Ackerman W. Verrucous carcinoma of the oral cavity. Surgery 1948; 23: 670-678.

[8]   Schwartz RA. Verrucous carcinoma of the skin and mucosa. J Am Acad Dermatol 1995; 32: 1-21.

[9]   Calender TA. Verrucous carcinoma of the head and neck.Bobby R. Alford Department of Otolaryngology- Head and Neck Surgery; 2009. Available at: www.bcn.edu/oto/grand/92891.html.

[10]   Murrah VA, Batsak JG. Proliferative verrucous leukoplakia and verrucous hyperplasia. Ann Otol Rhinol Laryngol 1994; 103: 660-663.

[11]   Shafer WG, Hine MK, Levy BM. A text book of oral pathology. Philadelphia, WB: Saunders Company, 1983. Benign and malign tumors of the oral cavity, pp.127-1130.

[12]   Spiro RH. Verrucous carcinoma, then and now. Amer J Surgery 1998; 176(5): 393-397.

[13]   Kolbusz, RV, Goldberg LH. Verrucous carcinoma of the oral cavity. Int J Dermatol 1994; 33: 618-622.

[14]   Shear M, Pinborg JJ. Verrucous hyperplasia of the oral mucosa. Cancer 1980; 46: 1855-1862.

[15]   Schwade JG, Wara WM, Dedo HH, Philips TL. Radiolucency for verrucous carcinoma. Radiology 1976; 120: 677-679.

[16]   Burns HP, van Nostrand AWP, Bryce DP. Verrucous carcinoma of the larynx. Management by radiotherapy and surgery. Ann Oto Rhino Laryngol 1976; 85: 538-543.

[17]   Aytekin A, Ay A, Okumus Y, Aytekin O. Reconstruction of an oral cavity defect resulting from verrucous carcinoma with a prefabricated parietal galeal flap. Annals of Plastic Surgery 2003; 50(1)106-107.

[18]   Oliveira D, Moraes R, Filho J, Landman G, Kowalski L. Oral verrucous carcinoma a retrospective study in Sao Paulo Region, Brazil. Clinical Oral Investigations 2006; 10(3): 205-209.

[19]   Keen WW. The surgical operations on President Cleveland. 1917. George W. Jacobs & Co. Philadelphia.

[20]   O'Connell JC. Becoming Cape Cod. 2002: University Press of New England: Hanover and London.

[21]   Health Media Lab. Grover Cleveland (1885-1889), (1893-1897) The Secret Operation. When the president is the patient; 2009. Available at: www.healthmedialab.com/html/president/cleveland.html.

[22]   Maloney W. Surreptitious surgery on Long Island Sound: the oral cancer surgeries of President Grover Cleveland. NY State Dent J 2010 Jan; 176: 42-45.

CHAPTER 17

The Asthma of President Calvin Coolidge

Abstract: Calvin Coolidge was an active, outdoor-type boy until he received his childhood diagnosis of asthma. This diagnosis had a very deep effect on the development of his personality. He grew up trying to avoid stressful or strenuous circumstances in order to not bring on the symptoms of his asthma. Asthma is a respiratory condition which many individuals throughout the world suffer with on a daily basis. Fortunately, individuals with asthma can lead very active and full lives today. The path chosen by 'Silent Cal' was reflected in his actions, or lack thereof, during his years as president of the United States.

Keywords: Allergen, allergies, asthma, coughing, dental examinations, fissure sealants, gingivitis, heart attack, oral candidiasis, Silent Cal, sneezing, stock market, tooth enamel.

PRESIDENT CALVIN COOLIDGE

Asthma shaped every aspect of Coolidge's personality. He chose to excel at politics. He worked his way up to the upper levels of Massachusetts politics and eventually became the 30th president of the United States. His devotion to leading a passive life was very obvious during Coolidge's years in the White House during which he would sleep for up to 11 hours per day [1].

Calvin Coolidge was born on July 4, 1872 in the village of Plymouth Notch, Vermont. The family lived in a house which was attached to the local general store and post office. The house and barns of his mother's family, the Moors, stood across the street [2].

The younger John Coolidge was a slight and slender youth who tried to avoid vigorous physical activity. His voice had a crackling quality about it. He started to develop symptoms of sneezing, coughing, and nasal mucous secretions.

Coolidge was beset by an attack of bronchitis which caused him to delay his enrollment at Amherst College for a year [3]. Once he arrived in college he dropped the suffix, Jr., and started to be known simply as Calvin Coolidge. After college graduation Coolidge practiced law in Northampton, Massachusetts before entering a life in politics. He was very successful and eventually became vice-president of the United States.

One morning, in August of 1923, he was vacationing in Vermont when he was awakened at 2:30 in the morning by his father with the news that President Warren Harding had unexpectedly died and that he was the new president of the United States. His father, a notary, administered the presidential oath of office using the family bible [4].

Coolidge's main form of exercise during his presidency was walking. He and his physician managed his asthma by breathing chlorine which was released into the air in a closed room [5].

In the summer of 1924, Coolidge's son, Calvin Jr., died of an infection [6]. The President never fully recovered from this loss.

Mrs. Coolidge wrote, in June of 1928, that the President was "having quite a lot of trouble with his asthma" [7] and that he "took his 'spray' along in the car" [8]. His asthmatic symptoms grew worse [3]. Coolidge decided against running for the White House in the next election as he was, at this point, using his spray every night to relieve his shortness of breath [3]. Herbert Hoover became the 31st president of the United States on March 4, 1929. Only seven months later, on October 24, 1929, the stock market crashed ushering in the Great Depression.

Coolidge suffered from a number of physical ailments after he left the White House. He had a rapid pulse rate, shortness of breath and gastrointestinal issues. He also experienced multiple asthmatic episodes. He started to experience extreme fatigue during the first week of 1933. On January 5, 1933 Coolidge passed away in Northampton, Massachusetts. The cause of death was a heart attack.

ASTHMA

Asthma is a chronic disease in which the airways of the lungs become inflamed and narrowed. It affects all races and ethnic groups. In America, 7% of the population has asthma [9-12]. Before puberty, boys are slightly more affected than girls. This trend reverses itself after puberty [9]. Worldwide, there are 300 million individuals living with asthma needing 500,000 hospitalizations each year for asthma-related incidents [13].

Individuals suffering from asthma may experience coughing, shortness of breath, chest tightness, and wheezing [14, 15] (Table **4**).

Table 4.   **Warning Signs of a Mild Asthmatic Episode**

-frequent cough
-shortness of breath
-tired or weak when exercising
-moody
-changes in peak expiratory flow
-sneezes
-runny nose
-sore throat
-congestion

THE DEVASTATING EFFECTS OF COOLIDGE'S PASSIVE PERSONALITY

As with other famous individuals, President Coolidge's medical life not only affected his personal life but, also his public persona. From a young age Coolidge made a conscious effort to deal with the fear of his asthma and the possible physical effects it might have on him by being an incredibly passive person and avoiding the stressful situations of life which so many other individuals throw themselves into in a headlong manner.

As Coolidge matured into an adult, his personality had taken shape and his passive demeanor now flowed forth naturally from him. Politics, and particularly the presidency of the United States, is not the place for an individual who is unwilling to take charge when necessary.

Coolidge stood by idly while the groundworks for the Great Depression were being laid. Unfortunately, many Americans and individuals worldwide would suffer the effects of Coolidge avoiding the difficult issues which true leaders have to manage whether they like it or not.

REFERENCES

[1]   McCoy DR. Calvin Coolidge: The Quiet President. New York: Macmillan 1967, 408-409.
[2]   Alen MGF. Calvin Coolidge. 2002; Enslow Publishers, Inc. Berkley Heights, NJ.
[3]   Cohen SG. Asthma among the famous. Allergy and Asthma Proc Jan-Feb 1998; 19 (1): 31-57.
[4]   The White House. Calvin Coolidge. 2010. Available at: http://www.whitehouse.gov/about/presidents/calvincoolidge.
[5]   Schaeffer JI. Faces of asthma. 2010. available at: http:// www.breatheeasyplayhard.com/pg/jsp/general/jsp/general/faces.jsp?faces=4.
[6]   Davidson Jr T, Conor KM. The impairment of presidents Pierce and Coolidge after traumatic bereavement. Comprehensive Psychiatry 2008; 49: 413-419.
[7]   Dictionary of American biography, s.v. Coolidge, Calvin. Starr HE, (Ed) New York: Scribner's, 1944, Suppl 1: 191-199.
[8]   McCoy DR. Calvin Coolidge: The Quiet President. New York: Macmillan, 1967, 389-390.
[9]   Fanta CH. Asthma. N Engl J Med 2009; 360(10): 1002-1014.
[10]   The state of asthma in america: asthma in america survey. 2009. Available at: http://www.asthmainamerica.com.
[11]   Expert Panel Report 3: Guidelines for the Diagnosis and Management of Asthma. Bethesda, MD: National Heart, Lung, and blood Institute, August 2007. (NIH publication no. 07-4051). 2009. Available at: http://nhlbi.nih.gov/guidelines/asthma/asthgdln.pdf.
[12]   Beasley R. The Global burden of asthma report. In: Global Initiative for asthma (GINa). 2009. available at: http://www.ginasthma.org.
[13]   Medical News Today. Updated NIH guidelines offer valuable information on asthma diagnosis and management. 2010. available at: http://www.medicalnewstoday.com/ar ticles /81140.php.
[14]   National Heart, Lung, and Blood Institute. What is asthma? 2010. Available at: http://www.nhlbi.nih.gov/health/dci/Diseases/asthma/asthma_WhatIs.html.
[15]   Cleveland Clinic. Symptoms of asthma. 2010. Available at: http:// my.clevelandclinic.org/disorders/asthma/hic_symptoms_of_asthma.aspx.

CHAPTER 18

An Analysis of the Theory that President Abraham Lincoln Suffered from an Undiagnosed Genetic Disorder

Abstract: Multiple endocrine neoplasia, type 2B is an autosomal dominant hamartoneoplastic syndrome which is caused by a heterozygous mutation in the RET gene located on chromosome 10g11. It is characterized by the development of multiple mucosal neuromas. Bumps which are glistening in appearance form along the tongue, lips, and lining of the mouth. An analysis of the physical characteristics of Abraham Lincoln has led researchers to recently theorize that he had multiple endocrine neoplasia, type 2B.

Keywords: American civil war, assassination, DNA, dura mater, fatigue, fibrillin, Ford's Theater, marfan's syndrome, medullary thyroid carcinoma, Mortality, multiple endocrine neoplasia, mutant.

ABRAHAM LINCOLN

Abraham Lincoln had the most humble of origins. He became both beloved and despised by his fellow countrymen during his lifetime. His life was tragically snuffed out by an assassin's bullet at the culmination of the defining period of his life- the American Civil War.

This simple yet complex man was be the guiding force behind the will of the Northern, or Union, states to prevent the dissolution of the nation described his early days [1], "I was born February 12, 1809, in Hardin County, Kentucky. My parents were both born in Virginia, of undistinguished families- second families, perhaps I should say. My mother, who died in my tenth year, was of a family of the name of Hanks ... My father ... removed from Kentucky to ... Indiana, in my eighth year ... It was a wild region, with many bears and other wild animals still in the woods. There I grew up ... Of course when I came of age I did not know much. Still somehow, I could read, write, and cipher ... but that was all" [2].

In December 1816 young Lincoln moved with his family to a three-sided shelter on Pigeon Creek sixteen miles north of the Ohio River because of the uncertainty of Kentucky land titles. Lincoln tried various jobs over the years and discovered his own likes and dislikes. Among his blossoming passions was a love for politics. In 1832 Lincoln ran for his first political office and lost. However, he was not deterred and won two years later [3].

In 1847 Lincoln entered into Washington politics for the first time. In the mid-1850's Lincoln left the Whig party to help found a new American political party-the Republican party. At this point Lincoln had his sights set on a seat in the United States Senate. This campaign will always be remembered more for his performances in a series of debates against Stephen Douglass than the fact that Lincoln eventually lost the 1858 senatorial election [4].

Abraham Lincoln was elected President of the United States in 1860 with the storm clouds of war rising over both the North and South of the United States. Lincoln was a staunch supporter of preserving the Union at, literally, any cost. There would be no negotiations on this point.

On April 12, 1861 Confederate or Southern forces, under the leadership of General P.G.T. Beauregard, fired on the sea fort of Fort Sumter in Charleston Harbor. These were the first shots of the American Civil War. By the next afternoon the bars and stars were flying within the fort.

The war was raged on for the next few years with one indecisive battle after another. The Confederate States of America would have their best chance at ultimate victory in July of 1863 when the troops of General Robert E. Lee would meet the Union troops of General George Meade in the wheatfields and dusty ridges, devilish dens and craggy hilltops of the, until then, peaceful and quiet western Pennsylvania town of Gettysburg. No better words could be ever written to describe the events [5] of the third and final day of the battle, July 3, than those of William Faulkner in 'Intruder in the Dust', "For every southern boy fourteen years old, not once but whenever he wants it, there is the instant when it's still not yet two o'clock on that July afternoon in 1863, the brigades are in position behind the rail fence, the guns are laid and ready in the woods and the furled flags are already loosened to break out and Pickett himself with his long oiled ringlets and his hat in one hand probably and his sword in the other looking up the hill waiting for Longstreet to give the word and it's all in the balance, it hasn't happened yet, it hasn't even begun yet, it not only hasn't begun yet but there is still time for it not to begin against that position and those circumstances ... that moment doesn't need even a fourteen year-old boy to think This time. Maybe this time with all this much to lose and all this much to gain: Pennsylvania, Maryland, the world, the gold dome of Washington itself ... [6]."

The Southern assault, which became known in the history books as Pickett's Charge, was a disaster for the Confederates as one after another brave Southern man fell. Although the war did not end that day, the eventual outcome of the war was determined as was the future of the Southern way of life which Margaret Mitchell would eloquently, yet somberly, describe years later as being "gone with the wind" [7].

On April 14, 1865 the man that saved the Union was assassinated at Ford's Theater only blocks from the White House as he and his wife attended a play, 'Our American Cousin'.

It is almost like Lincoln's favorite poem, William Knox's 'Mortality' [8], was written about his very own life, "O why should the spirit be proud! Like a fast flitting meteor, a fast flying cloud, a flash of the lightning, a break of the wave- he passes from life to his rest in the grave".

MULTIPLE ENDOCRINE NEOPLASIA, TYPE 2B

Multiple endocrine neoplasia, type 2B (MEN2B) is an autosomal dominant syndrome [9]. It is caused, in 95% of the cases, by a single amino acid substitution in the RET protein. Mucosal neuromas and a marfanoid habitus are present in almost 100% of MEN2B cases. Medullary thyroid carcinoma is found in over 95% of the cases while pheochromocytomas are present in about half of all MEN2B cases [10].

This disorder was initially described by Wagenmann [11] and Froboese [12]. 50% of cases of MEN2B arise *de novo* [13]. Both inherited and *de novo* MEN2B share in common a single identical point with a mutation in the catalytic core of the tyrosine kinase domain of RET [14]. In the inherited form the mutant RET allele is usually of paternal origin [15-17].

Surgery is a treatment modality in many individuals with MEN2B. Adrenalectomy is performed prior to thyroidectomy in those individuals who have been diagnosed with pheochromocytoma. This is done prior to a thyroidectomy to avoid an intraoperative catecholamine crisis [18]. It is advisable to screen for pheochromocytoma in individuals with MEN2B even if no symptoms are present. The physical examination should check for elevated blood pressure, an abdominal mass, and elevations of catecholamine levels in blood and/or urine [19].

LINCOLN'S MEDICAL HISTORY

"The eyelids and surrounding parts of the face were greatly ecchymosed and the eyes somewhat protuberant from effusion of blood into the orbits.

There was a gunshot wound on the head around which the scalp was greatly thickened by hemorrhage into its tissues. The ball entered through the occipital bone about one inch to the left of the median line and just above the left lateral sinus, which it opened. It then penetrated the dura mater, passed through the left posterior lobe of the cerebrum, entered the left lateral ventricle and lodged in the white matter of the cerebrum just above the anterior portion of the left corpus striatum, where it was found.

The wounds in the occipital bone were quite smooth, circular in shape, with beveled edges. The opening through the internal table was larger than that through the external table. The track of the ball was full of clotted blood and contained several little fragments of bone with a small piece of the ball near its external orifice. The brain around the track was pultaceous and livid from capillary hemorrhage into its substance. The ventricles of the brain were full of clotted blood. A thick clot beneath the dura mater coated the right cerebral lobe.

There was a smaller clot under the dura mater of the left side. But little blood was found at the base of the brain. Both the orbital plates of the frontal bone were fractured and the fragments pushed upwards towards the brain. The dura mater over these fractures was uninjured. The orbits were gorged with blood.

Your obedient servant,

E.J.J. Woodward" [20-22]

The above words describe the findings of the physicians who performed the autopsy on Abraham Lincoln. The interest of scientists and historians in the medical condition of Lincoln did not end with his autopsy. For an individual who died as a result of an assassin's bullet, Abraham Lincoln's medical history has certainly received a large amount of attention and interest from medical historians. The range of medical ailments which Lincoln is speculated to have had during his lifetime is vast. Some of these have included Marfan's syndrome, psychiatric disorders, and various neurological disorders.

Dr. John Sotos recently posited in his book [23] that Lincoln may have had a very rare, cancer-causing genetic disorder- MEN2B. This theory seems to be very plausible. Lincoln had many signs and symptoms which would support this argument.

In 1860 Lincoln began to lose significant weight as was noted by his contemporaries. As time marched on toward the fateful Good Friday of 1865, Lincoln started to develop headaches, cold feet, cold hands, exercise intolerance, and sweating. These findings are consistent with a diagnosis of pheochromocytoma which is a common cancer in MEN2B [24].

Other physical symptoms of Lincoln which support a diagnosis of MEN2B include Lincoln's height, long limbs, big feet, leanness, high voice, fatigue, intermittently drooping eyelids, loose jointedness, and an asymmetry in his facial features [4]. These are known as marfanoid features. Therefore, obviously, it is easy to confuse Marfan's syndrome with MEN 2B. Many scientists have speculated through the past few decades that Lincoln had Marfan's syndrome. Marfan's syndrome is a genetic condition which affects one in 5,000 to 10,000 individuals in the population. It is a deadly disorder of connective tissue which involves a defect in a protein known as fibrillin. A usual fatal result of this disorder is the rupture of the aorta [25].

Whether Lincoln truly had MEN2B and not Marfan's syndrome or some other disorder could easily be proven by a DNA test. The test looks for the mutation on chromosome 10 in the gene known as RET which is responsible for causing MEN2B [26]. The problem, of course, is obtaining a sample of the deceased President's DNA. There are plenty of samples existing but, gaining access to them has proven difficult. Dr. Sotos, who first theorized that Lincoln had MEN2B, was recently denied in his request to examine a small piece of fabric by the board of the Grand Army of the Republic Museum and Library [27].

Other researchers have speculated that Lincoln might have had spinocerebellar ataxia type 5 or SCA 5. It is a degenerative disease which has been found in 300 descendants of relatives of Lincoln [28]. Like MEN2B, any theory stating that Lincoln had SCA5 can only be proven by DNA testing. Scientists will have to rely on those boards which control the artifacts to allow them to test as Lincoln's body is presently inaccessible. Many years after his death, Lincoln was reburied in an 8 cubic foot block of concrete encased in iron bars. This was done in an effort to prevent future grave-robbing attempts [29].

Army surgeon Edward Curtis' words vividly describe and transport the reader back to the autopsy room: "The room...contained but little furniture: a large, heavily curtained bed, a sofa or two, bureau, wardrobe, and chairs....Seated around the room were several general officers and some civilians, silent or conversing in whispers, and to one side, stretched upon a rough framework of boards and covered only with sheets and towels, lay—cold and immovable—what but a few hours before was the soul of a great nation. The Surgeon General was walking up and down the room when I arrived and detailed me the history of the case. He said that the President showed most wonderful tenacity of life, and, had not his wound been necessarily mortal, might have survived an injury to which most men would succumb....Dr. Woodward and I proceeded to open the head and remove the brain down to the track of the ball. The latter had entered a little to the left of the median line at the back of the head, had passed almost directly forward through the center of the brain and lodged. Not finding it readily, we proceeded to remove the entire brain, when, as I was lifting the latter from the cavity of the skull, suddenly the bullet dropped out through my fingers and fell, breaking the solemn silence of the room with its clatter, into an empty basin that was standing beneath. There it lay upon the white china, a little black mass no bigger than the end of my finger—dull, motionless and harmless, yet the cause of such mighty changes in the world's history as we may perhaps never realize.... Silently, in one corner of the room, I prepared the brain for weighing. As I looked at the mass of soft gray and white substance that I was carefully washing, it was impossible to realize that it was that mere clay upon whose workings, but the day before, rested the hopes of the nation. I felt more profoundly impressed than ever with the mystery of that unknown something which may be named 'vital spark' as well as anything else, whose absence or presence makes all the immeasurable difference between an inert mass of matter owning obedience to no laws but those covering the physical and chemical forces of the universe, and on the other hand, a living brain by whose silent, subtle machinery a world may be ruled. The weighing of the brain...gave approximate results only, since there had been some loss of brain substance, in consequence of the wound, during the hours of life after the shooting. But the figures, as they were, seemed to show that the brain weight was not above the ordinary for a man of Lincoln's size." [21, 30] Dr. Curtis almost seemed to have been expecting to have found that Lincoln's brain was greater in size than the average man.

REFERENCES

[1]   Maher B. What Lincoln had. Nature. November 30, 2007.
[2]   The White House. Abraham Lincoln Accessed on September 27, 2013. Available at: http://www.whitehouse.gov/about/presidents/abrahamlincoln.
[3]   American National Biography Online. American national Biography Online: Lincoln, Abraham. Accessed on: October 31, 2013. Available at: http://www.anb.org/articles/ 04/04-00631.html.
[4]   Miller Center. American President: Abraham Lincoln (1809-1865). Accessed on October 29, 2013. Available at: http://millercenter.org/president/lincoln/essays/ biography/print
[5]   Accessed on April 24, 2014. Available at: http://www.muse.jhu.edu.muse.resources.apu.edu.

[6]   Faulkner W. Intruder in the Dust. Paperback, Vintage Classics, 247 pages; 1948.

[7]   Mitchell M. Gone With the Wind.1937; Macmillan, New York; 1037 pages.

[8]   Knox W. Mortailty.

[9]   Accessed on April 24, 2014. Available at: http://www.medigle.de/rw/diagnoses/multiple+
        endokrine+neoplasia+typ+2b.

[10]   The Merck Manual. Multiple endocrine neoplasia, type 2b (MEN, type 2b). accessed on
        October 31, 2013. Available at: http://www.merckmanuals.com/professional/ endocrine_
        and_metabolic_disorders/multiple_endocrine_neoplasia-men_syndromes/multiple_endocrin
        e_neoplasia_type_2b_men_2b.html.

[11]   Wagenmann A. Multiple neurome des auges und der Zunge. Ber. Dtsch. Ophthal. 43: 282-
        285, 1922.

[12]   Froboese C. Das aus markhaltigen nervenfascern bestehende gangliezellenlose echte
        neurom in rankenformzugleich ein beitrag zu den nervosen Geschwulsten der zunge und
        des augenlides. Virchows Arch. A Path. Anat. 240: 312-327, 1923.

[13]   Carlson KM, Dou S, Chi D, Scavarda N, Toshima K, Jackson CE, Wells SA Jr,
        Goodfellow PJ, Donis-Keller H. Single missense mutation in the tyrosine kinase catalytic
        domain of the RET protooncogene is associated with multiple endocrine neoplasia type 2B.
        Proc. Nat. Acad. Sci. 91: 1579-1583, 1994.

[14]   Carney JA, Go VLW, Sizemore GW, Hayles AB. Alimentary-tract ganglioneuromatosis: a
        major component of the syndrome of multiple endocrine neoplasia, type 2b. New Eng. J.
        Med. 295: 1287-1291, 1976.

[15]   DeSchryver-Kecskemeti K, Clouse RE, Goldstein MN, Gersell D, O'Neal L. Intestinal
        ganglioneuromatosis: a manifestation of overproduction of nerve growth factor? New Eng.
        J. Med. 308: 635-639, 1983.

[16]   Morrison PJ, Nevin NC. Multiple endocrine neoplasia type 2B (mucosal neuroma
        syndrome, Wagenmann-Froboese syndrome). J Med Genet. 1996 Sep; 33(9): 779-82.

[17]   Carlson KM, Bracamontes J, Jackson CE, Clark R, Lacroix A, Wells SA Jr, Goodfellow PJ.
        Parent-of-origin effects in multiple endocrine neoplasia type 2B. Am J Hum Genet. 1994
        Dec; 55(6): 1076-82.

[18]   Moline J and Eng C. Multiple endocrine neoplasia type 2. Accessed on November 1, 2013.
        Available at: http://www.ncbi.nlm.nih.gov/books/NBK1257/

[19]   The Children's Hospital of Philadelphia. Multiple endocrine neoplasia type 2. Accessed on
        October 1, 2013. Available at: http:www.chop.edu/services/oncology/ our=programs/hered
        itary-cancer-predisposition-program/genetic-syndromes-with-cancer-risks/multiple-endocrin
        e-neoplasia-type-2.html.

[20]   Dr. Woodward's autopsy report. April 15, 1865.

[21]   Friedman WA, Peace D. A Gunshot wound to the head- the case of Abraham Lincoln.
        Surgical Neurology May 2000; 53(5); 511-515.

[22]   National Museum of Health and Medicine. Accessed on April 24, 2014. Available at:
        www.medicalmuseum.mil/index.cfm?p=exhibits.lincoln.page_03

[23]   Sotos J. The Physical Lincoln (self-published), 2007.

[24]   Doctor Zebra. Health and medical history of President Abraham Lincoln. Accessed on:
        November 1, 2013. Available at: http://www.doctorzebra.com/prez/g16.htm

[25]   Brody JE. Marfan's Syndrome. New York Times. October 16, 2001.

[26]   Brown D. Is Lincoln earliest recorded case of rare disease? The Washington Post. November 26, 2007; page A08.

[27]   Bixler JP. DNA test could shed light on Lincoln's last days, doctor says. Accessed on November 20, 2013. Available at: http://www.cnn.com/2009/HEALTH/ 05/05/12/27/2006.

[28]   Associate Press. Disease may have caused Lincoln's 'clumsy gait.' 12/27/2006.

[29]   Maher B. What Lincoln had. Nature; 30 November 2007.

[30]   A letter from Edward Curtis to his mother.

CHAPTER 19

The Lazarus Syndrome

Abstract: The Lazarus Syndrome is a very real medical occurrence. It is known in medical terminology as delayed return of spontaneous circulation after cessation of cardiopulmonary resuscitation. It was first reported in the medical literature in 1982. One plausible mechanism for this event is dynamic hyperinflation of the lung causing positive end expiratory pressure. Some other medical investigators have suggested that a return of spontaneous circulation might be due to a delayed action of drugs which were administered during efforts to resuscitate the patient.

Keywords: Bethany, cardiac reperfusion, circulation, coronary artery, CPR, embolized endovascular plaque, expiratory pressure, Gospel, hyper-inflation, hyperkalemia, Lazarus syndrome, mechanisms of action, medical literature, neurological, phenomenon.

LAZARUS OF BETHANY

The masters of art throughout the ages have found the raising of Lazarus from his tomb a special subject for their work. Rembrandt, Caravaggio, and van Gogh were among these masters. The events surrounding the raising of Lazarus, by Jesus Christ, from the apparent dead has also been the subject of a multitude of authors, theologians, archeologists, and historians for the past two millenia. Now even medical professionals are studying the resurrection of Lazarus thus giving rise, so to speak, to the term 'Lazarus syndrome' or the 'Lazarus phenomenon'.

The death and apparent resurrection of Lazarus is described by St. John in his Gospel, "Now a man named Lazarus was sick. He was from Bethany, the village of Mary and her sister Martha ... the sisters sent word to Jesus, "Lord, the one you love is sick". When he heard this, Jesus said, "This sickness will not end in death. No, it is for God's glory so that God's Son may be glorified through it." Now Jesus loved Martha and her sister and Lazarus. So when He heard that Lazarus was sick, he stayed where he was two more days, and then he said to his disciples, "Let us go back to Judea." ... "Our friend Lazarus has fallen asleep; but I am going to wake him up." ... Jesus had been speaking of his death, but his disciples thought he meant natural sleep ... he told them plainly, "Lazarus is dead" ...On his arrival, Jesus found that Lazarus had already been in the tomb for four days ... Martha said to Jesus, "if you had been here, my brother would not have died" ... Jesus said to her, "Your brother will rise again." ... "I am the resurrection and the life. The one who believes in me will live, even though they die; and whoever lives by believing in me will never die" ... "Where have you laid him?" ... Jesus wept ... Jesus called in a loud voice, "Lazarus, come out!" The dead man came out, his hands and feet wrapped with strips of linen, and a cloth around his face [1-3]."

Not much is known of the circumstances of the life of Lazarus after his resurrection. However, there are numerous mythologies concerning this period. The tradition of the Eastern Orthodox Church states that he fled to Cyprus and was appointed the first bishop of Kition while others believe that he became the first bishop of Marseilles. Today, the Orthodox Church and the Byzantine Catholic Church commemorate Lazarus on Lazarus Saturday which is the day before Palm Sunday [3]. The Roman Catholic Church observes his memorial on July 29 which is the same day as his sister Martha's memorial [4].

THE LAZARUS SYNDROME

The Lazarus syndrome is a rare phenomenon. However, it is most probably not as rare as it is thought to be. It is likely very underreported in the scientific and medical literature for various reasons which are beyond the scope of this eBook.

The Lazarus syndrome is, without question, a real medical occurrence. It is known in medical terminology as delayed return of spontaneous circulation after cessation of cardiopulmonary resuscitation. This syndrome was first described in the medical literature in 1982. In 1983 Bray first associated this phenomenon with the resurrected biblical individual [5, 6]. There have only been less than 50 cases of this syndrome reported in the medical literature [5-32].

In individuals who have experienced this medical phenomenon, all efforts at performing cardiopulmonary resuscitation (CPR) have been terminated. Within approximately 10 minutes after the cessation of CPR a very unexpected return of spontaneous circulation is observed. There is a case reported where a young man was declared dead and a pulse was found 30 minutes after his death was declared [32]. Many of these patients eventually recovered fully and were discharged from the hospital with no neurological sequelae.

Some proposed theoretical mechanisms of action are 1) a dynamic hyperinflation of the lung causing increased positive end expiratory pressure; 2) a delayed action of drugs which were used during CPR; and 3) a result of hyperkalemia [33]. Another proposed mechanism is that cardiac reperfusion can result from a dislodging of embolized endovascular plaque from the coronary artery [20, 24].

Due to the Lazarus syndrome it is certainly advisable for healthcare professionals to wait at least 10 minutes after apparent death for the death of an individual to be formally declared.

REFERENCES

[1]   Bible Gateway. The Death of Lazarus. Accessed on March 17, 2014. Available at: www.biblegateway.com/passage/?search=John+11.

[2]   Accessed on April 25, 2014. Available at: http://www.jesusleroc.com/pub/weekly-devotion-archives-detail.php?id=506

[3]   Catholic Online. St. Lazarus of Bethany. Accessed on September 28, 2013. Available at: http://www.catholic.org/saints/saint.php?saint_id=4220

[4]   Martyrolgium Romanum 420 (edito altera 2005).

[5]   Bray JG. The Lazarus phenomenon revisited. Anesthesiology 1993; 78: 991.

[6]   Linko K, Honkavaara P, Salmenpera M. Recovery after discontinued cardiopulmonary resuscitation. Lancet 1982; 1: 106-107.

[7]   Letellier N, Coulomb F, Lebec C, Brunnet JM. Recovery after discontinued cardiopulmonary resuscitation. Lancet 1982; 1: 1019.

[8]   Klockgether A, Kontokollias JS, Geist J, Schoenneich A. Monitoring in Rettungsdienst. Notarzt 1987; 3: 85-88.

[9]   Rosengarten PL, Tuxen DV, Dziukas L, Scheinkestel C, Merret K, Bowes G. Circulatory arrest induced by intermittent positive pressure ventilation in a patient with severe asthma. Anaesth Intensive Care 1991; 19: 118-121.

[10]   Skulberg A. Criteria of death and time of death- do Norwegian physicians follow laws and regulations? [Norwegian]. Tidsskr Nor Lageforen 1991; 111: 3310-3311.

[11]   Rogers PL, Schlichtig R, Miro A, Pinsky M. Auto-PEEP during CPR: an 'occult' cause of electromechanical dissociation? Chest 1991; 99: 492-493.

[12]   Martens P, Vandekerckhove Y, Mullie A. Restoration of spontaneous circulation after cessation of cardiopulmonary resuscitation. Lancet 1993; 341: 841

[13]   Quick G, Bastani B. Prolonged asystolic hyperkalemic cardiac arrest with no neurological sequelae. Ann Emerg Med 1994; 24: 305-311.

[14]   Lapinsky SE, Leung RS. Auto-PEEP and electromechanical dissociation. NEJM 1996; 335: 674.

[15]   Voelckel W, Kroesen G. Unexpected return of cardiac action after termination of cardiopulmonary resuscitation. Resuscitation 1996; 32: 27-29.

[16]   Gomes E, Araujo R, Abrunhosa R, Rodrigues G. Two successful cases of spontaneous recovery after cessation of CPR. Resuscitation 1996; 31: 40.

[17]   Mutzbauer TS, Stahl W, Lindner KH. Compression-Decompression (ACD)-CPR. Prehosp Disaster Med 1997; 12: S21.

[18]   Fumeaux T, Borgeat A, Cuenoud PF, Erard A, de Werra P. Survival after cardiac arrest and severe acidosis (pH 6.54). Intensive Care Med 1997; 23: 594.

[19]   Maleck WH, Piper SN, Triem J, Boldt J, Zittel FU. Unexpected return of spontaneous circulation after cessation of resuscitation (Lazarus phenomenon). Resuscitation 1998; 39: 125-128.

[20]   Frolich MA. Spontaneous recovery after discontinuation of intraoperative cardiopulmonary resuscitation: case report. Anesthesiology 1998; 89: 1252-1253.

[21]   MacGillivray RG. Spontaneous recovery after discontinuation of cardiopulmonary resuscitation. Anesthesiology 1999; 91: 585-586.

[22]   Bradbury N. Lazarus phenomenon: another case? Resuscitation 1999; 41: 87.

[23]   Adhiyaman V, Sundaram R. The Lazarus phenomenon. J R Coll Phys Edin 2002; 32: 9-13.

[24]   Ben-David B, Stonebraker VC, Hersham R, Frost CL, Williams HK. Survival after failed intraoperative resuscitation: a case of 'Lazarus Syndrome'. Anesth Analg 2001; 92: 690-692.

[25]   Abdullah RS. Restoration of circulation after cessation of positive pressure ventilation in a case of 'Lazarus Syndrome'. Anesth Analg 2001; 93: 241.

[26]   Walker A, McClelland H, Brenchley A. Lazarus phenomenon following recreational drug use. Emerg Med J 2001; 18: 74-75.

[27]   Maeda H, Fujita MQ, Zhu BL, *et al*. Death following spontaneous recovery from cardiopulmonary arrest in a hospital mortuary: 'Lazarus phenomenon' in a case of alleged medical negligence. Forensic Sci Int 2002; 127: 82-87.

[28]   Duck MH, Paul M, Wixforth J, Kammerer H. The Lazarus phenomenon. Spontaneous return of circulation after unsuccessful intraoperative resuscitation in a patient with a pacemaker (German). Anaesthesist 2003; 52: 413-418.

[29]   Casielles Garcia JL, Gonzalez Latorre MV, Fernadez Amigo N, *et al*. Lazarus phenomenon: spontaneous resuscitation (Spanish). Rev Esp Anestesiol Reanim 2004; 51: 390-394.

[30]   De Salvia A, Guardo A, Orrico M, De Leo D. A new case of Lazarus phenomenon? Forensic Sci Int 2004; 146: S13-15.

[31]   Al-Ansari MA, Abouchaleh NM, Hijazi MH. Return of spontaneous circulation after cessation of cardiopulmonary resuscitation in a case of digoxin overdosage. Clinical Intensive Care 2005; 16: 179-181.

[32]   Monticelli F, Bauer N, Meyer HJ. Lazarus phenomenon. Current resuscitation standards and questions for the expert witness 9German). Rechtmedizin 2006; 16: 57-63.

[33]   MailOnline. Lazarus syndrome man pronounced dead comes back to life for two days. Accessed on October 4, 2013. Available at: http:www.dailymail.co.uk/news/ article-1192283/Lazarus-syndrome-man-pronounced-dead-comes-life-days.html.

[33]   Adhiyaman V, Adhiyaman S, Sundaram R. The Lazarus phenomenon. J R Soc Med. 2007 December; 100(12): 552-557.

CHAPTER 20

Tuberculosis: The Cause of the Early Death of John Keats

Abstract: John Keats was an English Romantic poet born in the late 1700's. Among his better known works are 'Ode on a Grecian Urn' and 'Ode to a Nightingale'. Keats suffered a series of hemorrhages in 1820 and died at the age of 25 from tuberculosis. Tuberculosis is a potentially fatal disease caused by a bacterium known as Mycobacterium tuberculosis. It usually attacks the lungs but can also affect other parts of the body such as the brain, kidneys, and spine.

Keywords: Brain, chills, coughing, droplets, Enfield Academy, fatigue, fever, Licentiate of the Society of Apothecaries, night sweats, spinal column, tuberculosis, weight loss.

JOHN KEATS

John Keats was born in Finsbury Pavement, near London, on October 31, 1795. Keats was born as the eldest son of a stablekeeper and had three brothers and a sister. His early years were relatively unstable as his father died when Keats was only eight years old and his mother remarried within the year. She quickly left her new husband and returned to her own mother, with her children, to live [1].

Young John's mother died of tuberculosis when he was only 15. John had been studying at Enfield Academy since shortly after his father's death. At Enfield, his burgeoning interest in literature was being nurtured by the headmaster, John Clarke. Unfortunately for Keats, his grandmother turned over control of the family's finances after John's mother's death to a London merchant, Richard Abbey [2]. Because of the financial turmoil, Keats had to withdraw from Enfield. However, he went on to study medicine at Guy's Hospital and obtained the Licentiate of the Society of Apothecaries in 1816.

On May 5, 1816 Keats' first poem, 'O Solitude! If I Must with Thee Dwell', was published in the Examiner. Shortly before his 21st birthday, Keats announced to close friends and colleagues, to the astonishment and ridicule of some, that he intended to make his living as a poet rather than in the medical profession [3].

After returning from a tour of Scotland and Northern England in the summer of 1818 to care for his brother who was suffering from tuberculosis, Keats met and fell in love with a woman named Fanny Brawne [4]. The two became engaged but, kept it a secret as Keats did not have the financial means to support a wife. It was not until many years after the poet's death that the public became aware that the two had been engaged. During the last years of his life, Keats published his third and best volume of poetry. This volume contained the unfinished 'Hyperion' which is considered to be amongst the greatest poetry ever written in the English language.

TUBERCULOSIS

Tuberculosis is a disease that has affected humans for thousands of years. The bacteria that causes tuberculosis, Mycobacterium tuberculosis, has been isolated in the spinal column of Egyptian mummies dating back to 2400 BCE [5].

Tuberculosis is spread person-to-person by one individual with infectious tuberculosis coughing or sneezing and another individual inhaling the bacterium-containing droplets. Individuals with tuberculosis in organs other than the lungs are rarely infectious [6].

Latent tuberculosis refers to the bacteria being present in an individual's body but causing no active symptoms and not being contagious. Active tuberculosis is when the affected individual shows signs of tuberculosis infection. This individual is contagious.

Signs and symptoms of active tuberculosis include cough, fatigue, night sweats, loss of appetite, unintentional weight loss, fever, and chills [7].

While the lungs are the most common organ affected by tuberculosis, other areas of the body may be the focal point of the infection. They are the brain, spine, and kidneys. Fortunately, today there are drugs which are very effective in treating tuberculosis. They include isoniazid, rifampin, ethambutol, and pyrazinamide [8].

The Tuberculosis Skin Test, also known as the Mantoux Test, is a very simple and painless way of determining if an individual has a latent tuberculosis infection.

Individuals who should have such a test are those that live or work in a nursing home, clinic, prison, hospital or homeless shelter; those who have HIV; individuals who are in close contact with someone who has active tuberculosis; and someone who has lived in a country where many people have tuberculosis [9].

THE TUBERCULOSIS OF JOHN KEATS

In June of 1818 Keats undertook a very strenuous walking tour of northern England and Scotland with his friend Charles Armitage Brown. After approximately two-thirds of the tour Keats started to complain of a sore throat. Most scholars agree that he acquired tuberculosis some time prior to the walking tour but, the strain of the feat brought on the first symptoms of tuberculosis [10, 11].

The winter of 1818 was marked by confusion and depression for Keats. He continued to prepare his poetry for publication despite an increase in both bodily and mental symptoms. A fierce hemorrhagic episode occurred in February of 1820 during which blood was coming from his mouth. Other similar episodes followed in June and July [12].

Keats' health, having deteriorated even more, left for Rome in November of 1820 in hopes that Rome's weather might have some positive effect on his health.

He was accompanied by a young painter, Joseph Severn [13]. It was in Severn's arms that Keats died on February 23, 1821. It was a great relief of suffering for Keats. His last words spoke to this- "... I shall die easy- don't be frightened- be firm, and thank God it has come! [14]"

In a letter to Keats' sister shortly after his death, Fanny Brawne wrote, "I am patient, resigned, very resigned. I know my Keats is happy, I know my Keats is happy, happier a thousand times than he could have been here ... you do not, you never can know how much he has suffered. So much that I do believe, were it in my power I would not bring him back. All that grieves me now is that I was not with him, and so near it as I was ... he at least was never deceived about his complaint, though the Doctors were ignorant and unfeeling enough to send him to that wretched country to die, for it is now known that his recovery was impossible before he left us, and he might have died here with so many friends to soothe him and me with him. All we have to console ourselves with is the great joy he felt that all his misfortunes were at an end [14]."

REFERENCES

[1]   John-Keats.com. Biography. Accessed on September 27, 2013. Available at: http://www.john-keats.com/

[2]   Bio. true story. John Keats. biography. Accessed on October 24, 2013. Available at: http://www.biography.com/people/john-keats-9361568.

[3]   Smith H. John Keats: poet, patient, physician. Reviews of Infectious Diseases May- June 1984; 6(3): 390-404.

[4]   The Academy of American Poets. John Keats. Accessed on October 28, 2013. Available at: http://www.poets.org/poet.php/prm/PID/66

[5]   New Jersey Medical School Global Tuberculosis Institute. History of TB. Accessed on December 24, 2013. Available at: http://globaltb.njms.rutgers.edu/tbhistory.htm

[6]   Tuberculosis Clinical Diagnosis and Management of Tuberculosis, and Measures for Its Prevention and Control; NICE Clinical Guidelines, No. 117. London: National Institute for Health and Clinical Excellence (UK): March 2011.

[7]   Mayo Clinic. tuberculosis. Accessed on December 23, 2013. Available at: http://www.mayoclinic.com/health/tuberculosis/D500372/DSECTION=symptoms

[8]   Centers for Disease Control and Prevention. Tuberculosis (TB). Accessed on 12/25/13. Available at: http:www.cdc.gov/tb/topic/treatment/default.htm

[9]   Minnesota Department of Health. The TB Skin Test (Mantoux). Accessed on 12/26/13. Available at: http://www.health.state.mn.us/divs/idepc/diseases/tb/factsheets/tsteng.pdf

[10]   Smith H. The Strange case of Mr. Keats's tuberculosis. Clin Infect Dis 2004; 38(7): 991-993.

[11]   Walker C. Walking north with Keats. New Haven, CT: Yale University Press; 1992.

[12]   Sharp W. Life and Letters of Joseph Severn. London: Low, Marston, and Co.; 1892.

[13]   Lowell A. John Keats (New York & Boston: Houghton-Mifflin, 1925)

[14]   English History. Net. John Keats and Fanny Brawne. Accessed on January 28, 2014. Available at: http:englishhistory.net/keats/fannybrawne.html.

CHAPTER 21

The Huntington's Disease of Woody Guthrie

Abstract: Woody Guthrie was born on July 14, 1912 in Okemah, Oklahoma. Guthrie grew into a popular musician helping to usher in a generation of folk music. Guthrie exhibited various physical symptoms and was misdiagnosed on multiple occasions. Among these misdiagnoses were alcoholism and schizophrenia. The proper diagnosis of Huntington's Disease was eventually made. Huntington's Disease is an inherited degenerative disease which affects the nerve cells in the brain. It results in cognitive, movement, and psychiatric disorders.

Keywords: Abnormal eye movements, appetite, dystonia, gait, Huntington's Disease, indecisiveness, muscle rigidity, sleeping problems, spatial perception, speech, suicide.

WOODY GUTHRIE

On July 2, 1912 Woodrow Wilson, America's 28th president, received the Democratic Party's nomination for the presidency of the United States. 12 days later a baby boy was born in Okemah, Oklahoma and his parents named him after the politician. Little Woodrow Wilson Guthrie grew up to become a prolific songwriter traveling throughout America singing the songs of the poor and downtrodden, the worker and common man.

Young Woody was profoundly affected by his parents musical tendencies. Charles Guthrie taught his son various Scottish, Indian, and folk songs [1]. Woody's early years in Okemah also greatly influenced his opinions on life and, in turn, his future musical direction. Woody saw Okemah turn into a quintessential oil boom town overnight as oil was discovered nearby. Speculators and all sorts of businessmen came to town. However, eventually, the oil dried up just as quickly as it was discovered. This affected the town and its people in a myriad of ways. Even deeper than the financial mess that the oil speculators left the town in was the damage done to the collective psyche of the townspeople. Woody developed a great distrust of the nation's power brokers and businesses after seeing first hand how his town was abandoned when it ceased to provide financial profits to the outsiders.

Woody learned how to play the mandolin, guitar, fiddle, and harmonica and joined a musical group called the Corncob Trio which played songs by country music greats such as the Carter Family and Jimmie Rodgers [2].

At the start of World War II Woody moved to New York City and then joined the United States Merchant Marine in 1943. After leaving the Merchant Marine two years later, Woody married Marjorie Greenblatt Mazia. The couple had four children [3]. They would divorce as Woody would travel about leaving the care of the children to his wife. During this period Guthrie would write hundreds of songs as he led his vagabond life.

Woody's fame increased as his health declined. Guthrie influenced many future musicians ranging from Bob Dylan to Bruce Springsteen to John Mellencamp. Woody Guthrie was inducted into the Rock and Roll Hall of Fame in 1988.

HUNTINGTON'S DISEASE

Huntington's Disease is a genetic disorder which is caused by a genetic defect on chromosome 4. It usually affects individuals in their mid 30's and 40's [4]. Some signs and symptoms of Huntington's Disease are behavioral disturbances, irritability, paranoia, psychosis, facial movements, unsteady gait, head turning to shift eye position, sudden movement of extremities, slow and uncontrolled movements, confusion, loss of judgment, loss of memory, tremor, personality changes, and difficulty swallowing (Table **5**). Huntington's Disease was described by an American physician, George Huntington, in 1872. Dr. Huntington's father and grandfather were both also physicians. Huntington would often accompany his father to work, as a boy, and was fascinated by those patients who were affected by the yet unnamed neurological disorder. Dr. Huntington used his youthful observations and those of his father and grandfather to produce his seminal paper at the age of 21 [5-9].

At this time there is no cure for Huntington's Disease. However, there are a few medications available to relieve some of its symptoms [10, 11].

Table 5.   Signs and Symptoms of Huntington's Disease [1-3]

-sleeping problems
-lack of flexibility in behavior
-changes in appetite
-indecisiveness
-thoughts of suicide
-involuntary jerking
-dystonia
-muscle rigidity
-uncoordinated fine movement
-abnormal eye movements
-lack of self-awareness
-difficulty focusing
-difficulty learning
-difficulty processing thoughts
-sadness
-poor spatial perception
-lack of interest in normal activities
-social withdrawal
-difficulty planning
-inability to start a task
-impaired gait and balance
-difficulty swallowing
-difficulty with speech

THE ILLNESS OF WOODY GUTHRIE

Guthrie suffered for 15 years with Huntington's Disease. Despite living with the symptoms of Huntington's Disease for a long time, Guthrie was somehow extremely successful professionally having written over 1,400 songs throughout his career.

Guthrie himself best describes how the illness affected him in a song he wrote entitled 'Huntington's Chorea Blues', "I got this thing called chorea in my head / wanna walk but I fall down instead / folks say "Woody, he's drunk again" / but I haven't had a drink since I don't know when / besides ... I only drink when I'm alone ... or with somebody / my arms felt funny moving all the time / and sometimes my head didn't feel like mine / kept telling myself it was the Ballantine Ale / and them jugs of wine on the writing trail / I prefer a disease you can sober up from [12]."

Guthrie's health steadily declined through the 1950's and his physicians had trouble diagnosing his illness. Unfortunately for Guthrie, his ambiguous physical and psychological symptoms led him to be placed in a psychiatric institution. This was the usual course of events for individuals in the 1950's who were diagnosed with Huntington's Disease. Guthrie spent the final 12 years of his life in a psychiatric hospital where he would be visited often by his second wife and his children.

While at Greystone Park Psychiatric Hospital in New Jersey he was visited by a young admirer who travelled all the way from Minnesota to meet his idol. The young man's name was Bob Dylan.

Guthrie moved to Brooklyn State Hospital in 1961 and five years later to the Creedmoor Psychiatric Center in Queens, New York where he died on October 3, 1967 at the age of 55.

Woody's widow, Marjorie Guthrie was determined to help other families who suffered from Huntington's Disease. Marjorie placed a small ad in a New York City newspaper to reach out to other individuals. She eventually compelled President Jimmy Carter to form a Presidential Commission to study neurological diseases. A report was issued in 1977 which gave recommendations which were instrumental in finding effective treatments for Huntington's Disease [13].

REFERENCES

[1]   Woody Guthrie. Woody Guthrie's Biography. Accessed on January 1, 2014. Available at: http://www.woodyguthrie.org/biography/biography1.htm.
[2]   Rock and Roll Hall of Fame and Museum. Woody Guthrie biography. Accessed on November 23, 2013. Available at: http://rockhall.com/inductees/woody-guthrie/bio/.
[3]   Mayo Clinic. Huntington's disease. Accessed on 12/20/13. Available at: www.mayoclinic. com/health/huntingtons-disease/DS00401.
[4]   Lang A. Other movement disorders. In: Goldman L, Ausiello D, eds. Cecil Medicine. 23rd ed. Philadelphia, Pa: Saunders Elsevier; 2007: chap 434.
[5]   Jankovic J, Shannon KM. Movement disorders. In: Bradley WG, Daroff RB, Fenichel GM, Jankovic J, eds. Bradley: Neurology in Clinical Practice. 5th ed. Philadelphia, Pa: Butterworth-Heinemann Elsevier; 2008: chap 75.
[6]   Furtado S, and Suchowersky O.Huntington's disease: recent advances in diagnosis and management. Can J Neurol Sci 1995; 22: 5-12.

[7]   Haddad MS, and Cummings JL. Huntington's disease. Psychiatr Clin North Am 1997; 20: 791-807.

[8]   Harper PS, and Morris M, 1991. Introduction: a historical background. in Huntington's Disease, W.B. Saunders, London; pp. 1-35.

[9]   Huntington G, 1872. On chorea. Medical and Surgical Reporter 26: 320-321.

[10]   Nasir J, Goldberg YP, and Hayden MR, 1996. Huntington disease: new insights into the relationship between CAG expansion and disease. Hum. Mol. Genet. 5: 1431-1435.

[11]   Huntington's Disease Society of America. hsda: a leader in global hd research. Accessed on 12/31/13. Available at: http://www.hdsa.org/research/hsda-research.html

[12]   Molecular Anatomy Project. Huntington's Disease. Accessed on 12/14/13. Available at: http://maptest_rutgers.edu/drupal/?q=node/40/

[13]   The Official Woody Guthrie Website. Accessed on 12/12/13. Available at: http://www.woodyguthrie.org/thislandconcert/hsda.htm

CHAPTER 22

The Mowgli Syndrome

Abstract: Rudyard Kipling was an English author who was born in Bombay in 1865. He was awarded the Nobel Prize in literature in 1907. Kipling's 'The Jungle Book' is a collection of stories. The most popular character in these stories is Mowgli, a 'man cub', who is raised by wolves in the Indian jungle. The Mowgli syndrome refers to feral children who, during their developmental years, have lacked proper care or human contact.

Keywords: Baloo the Bear, Captain Holloway, Carrie Balestier, Dummerston, Vermont, feral, India, insomnia, Mowgli, social skills, wolf.

RUDYARD KIPLING

Rudyard Kipling was born on December 30,1865 to John and Alice Kipling in Bombay. At the age of 5 he was sent by his parents back to England to live with a foster family in Southsea [1]. The youthful Kipling was despondent in this English house of Captain Holloway and his wife. He would not let on to any of his classmates or family any hint of the horrors which occurred in this foster household. Kipling was often beaten by Mrs. Holloway. He later wrote, "Then the old Captain died, and I was sorry, for he was the only person in that house as far as I can remember who ever threw me a kind word" [2]. Kipling referred to the Holloway house as 'The House of Desolation'.

In 1881 Kipling went back to India to live with his parents in Lahore. At this point Kipling became editor of 'Civil and Military Gazette' and 'The Pioneer' [2]. Kipling was accepted by both his fellow Englishmen who were living in India and by the locals. This dual acceptance, combined with Kipling's insomnia, allowed the young writer to gain access to many places where Englishmen were usually not welcome. These included the local brothels and opium dens. His experiences from this period were collected into 'Plain Tales from the Hills' which became very popular in England [3].

Kipling went on to write travel essays. While traveling through the United States he met Mark Twain. This meeting influenced Kipling greatly.

In 1892 Kipling married Carrie Balestier and rented a farm in Dummerston, Vermont. In his Vermont home Kipling began to work on the 'Jungle Books'. Kipling also received many visitors at his Vermont home including Arthur Conan Doyle [4].

Kipling lived at this house which he named Naulakha from 1892 to 1896. The beautiful house overlooked the Connecticut River and was in the shape of a ship [5]. The desk at which Kipling wrote the 'Jungle Books' remains in the house today [6]. It was during these years at Naulakha that the couple's second child was born. Kipling became involved in an embarrassing dispute with his wife's family which prompted him to move back to England in 1896. A year later their son, John, was born.

Kipling would receive (and turn down) many awards during his life. In 1907 Kipling became the first author to accept the Nobel Prize for literature. Kipling passed away in 1936 and is interred at Westminster Abbey [7].

THE JUNGLE BOOK

The 'Jungle Book' [8] is Kipling's collection of short stories which were first published in magazines in 1894. It was followed by 'The Second Jungle Book' in 1895. 'The Jungle Book' gave the world many memorable characters including Mowgli, Rikki-Tikki the mongoose, Baloo the Bear, and Bagheera the black panther.

On first glance, 'The Jungle Book' is merely a playful book for children. Rather, it is filled with satire and political commentary concerning the British imperialistic period in India. 'The Jungle Book' examines various human relationships and qualities such as loyalty, courage, honor, and persistence.

Elsie Bambridge was the only one of Kipling's three children who survived him. She lived as a married woman in England. She died in 1977 with no children and left her 10,000 book library to Britain's National Trust. Scholars have presented various theories concerning the inspiration for Kipling's iconic book. The answer was very simply revealed in 2010 when librarians came across a first edition of 'Jungle Book' while cataloging her collection. Upon opening the book they were startled to find a note Kipling had written to his daughter, Josephine, who died in 1899 at the age of 6, "This book belongs to Josephine Kipling for whom it was written by her father, May 1894" [9].

THE MOWGLI SYNDROME

Mowgli is a character in Kipling's 'Jungle Book' stories. Mowgli was lost by his parents as a baby in the Indian jungle. He was saved and raised by a wolf family.

The Mowgli syndrome takes its name from Kipling's character. It refers to feral children. These children have not received any human nurturing during their formative years [10]. When found by humans, these feral children usually exhibit the behavior of the animals with which they were in contact [11] (Table **6**).

Table 6.   **Signs of Mowgli's Syndrome [9]**

-lack all social skills
-do not walk upright
-may have physical deformities
-will not wear clothes
-are not interested in human activity
-do not understand language
-can not learn or speak a language

The term 'Mowgli Syndrome' was originally coined by Wendy Doninger O'Flaherty in her 1995 book 'Other People's Myths: The Cave of Echoes' [12].

REFERENCES

[1]   The Kipling Society. Rudyard Kipling. Accessed on 9/25/13. Available at: http://www.kipling.org.uk/kip_fra.htm.
[2]   Kipling R. Something of Myself: For My Friends Known and Unknown. Doubleday, Doran and Company, Garden City (NY), 1937.
[3]   Bio.Com. Rudyard Kipling. Accessed on: 10/9/13. Available at: www.biography.com/people/rudyard_kipling-936558.
[4]   The European Graduate School. Rudyard Kipling. Accessed on October 8, 2013. Available at: http://www.egs.edu/library/rudyard-kipling/biography/.

[5]   Ring W. Scholars visit Vermont birthplace of 'The Jungle Book.' Accessed on October 12, 2013. Available at: http://www.burlingtonfreepress.com/viewart/20131007/ NEWS07/3100 70024/US-UK-Kipling-scholars-visit-author-s-Vthome.

[6]   Connecticut River Joint Commissions. Naulakha (Kipling House). Accessed on October 14, 2013. Available at: http://www.crjc.org/heritage/vo3-3.htm.

[7]   BBC. Rudyard Kipling. Accessed on 10/7/13. Available at: http://www.bbc.co.uk/ history/historic_figures/kipling_rudyard.shtml.

[8]   Kipling R. The Jungle Book Illustrated by Scott McKowen. New York: Sterling; 2007.

[9]   The New York Times. A Rare "Jungle Book" Resurfaces in Britain. April 11, 2010.

[10]   Social-Psych. Feral Children: Mowgli Syndrome. Accessed on 10/11/13. Available at: http://social-psych.net/feral-children-mowgli-syndrome/.

[11]   Stewart W. First picture of neglected 'Mowgli' girl, 5, who was raised by dogs. Accessed on 10/13/13. Available at: http://www.dailymail.co.uk/news/article-1188976/ First-picture-year-old-Mowgli-girl-Natasha-Mikhailova-barks-like-dog-parents-neglected- her.html.

[12]   Doninger W. Other People's Myths: The Cave of Echoes. The University of Chicago Press 1995.

CHAPTER 23

Temporal Lobe Epilepsy: The Possible Medical Cause of the Conversion of St. Paul

Abstract: St. Paul was an early Christian follower of Jesus. Paul was converted to Christianity in what has become known as the Damascus Road experience. Prior to his conversion Paul persecuted Christians. Seizures of temporal lobe epilepsy occur in individuals of any age. Hallucinations of voice, people, smell, taste and music may occur during a seizure. Some individuals experience temporal lobe epilepsy after meningitis or a head injury. There is speculation that St. Paul's conversion was a result of a temporal lobe epileptic seizure.

Keywords: Body posture, bright light, Damascus, epilepsy, fear, hallucinations, head injury, hypergraphia, hyperreligiosity, hyposexuality, meningitis, Saul, seizures.

ST. PAUL

The life and actions of Paul can be viewed as being his life's dichotomy. Paul was originally known by a different name- Saul. His life's journey began in what is now Turkey in a city called Tarsus between 1 and 10 A.D. Tarsus was a well-developed and prosperous city located within the boundaries of the Roman Empire [1].

Although little is known of Paul's personal early upbringing, it seems likely that he was a student of the great rabbi Gamaliel I in Jerusalem [1, 2]. Gamaliel was a prominent member of the highest tribune of the Jews and the first to whom the title 'Rabban' or 'our master' was given. Gamaliel was responsible for sparing the lives of St. Peter and the Apostles who continued to preach to the common people despite a direct prohibition against this activity by the Jewish authorities. Gamaliel, according to Christian ecclesiastical tradition, is said to have accepted the Christian belief while Christianity was in the earliest stages of its infancy. He was baptized into the Christian faith by St. Peter and St. John themselves. He remained a member of the powerful Sanhedrin in order to secretly help his now fellow Christians [3].

Saul himself was baptized as Paul after his Damascus Road experience and retreated to Arabia for three years to pray. Antioch would later become the center for Paul's evangelizing efforts. He gradually became accepted by the other apostles who were, at first, very skeptical of Paul's intentions. Paul went on to write fervently. Thirteen epistles in the New Testament are credited to Paul. In his letters, Paul wrote of the Last Supper and the final battle between good and evil [4].

In Christian tradition, Paul was executed in Rome in the mid-60's at Tre Fontane Abbey during the reign of Nero.

The Vatican has recently excavated the supposed tomb of Paul at the Basilica of Saint Paul Outside the Walls. Pope Benedict, in June of 2009, announced that a probe was inserted into the sarcophagus revealing incense, and purple and blue linen. Also bone fragments were discovered which were later radiocarbon dated to the first or second century. The sarcophagus was also inscribed in Latin which read when translated, "Paul Apostle Martyr" [5].

TEMPORAL LOBE EPILEPSY

Temporal lobe epilepsy is one of the most common forms of epilepsy. The temporal lobes are located on either side of one's skull just above the ears [6]. A person experiencing a temporal lobe seizure may experience a sudden emergence of old memories, hallucinations of voices, music, smells, or tastes. The individual might also experience feelings of unusual fear or joy [6].

The Russian novelist, Fyodor Dostoyevsky, described the effects of such a seizure from which he himself suffered in vivid detail in his novel 'The Idiot', "He remembered that during his epileptic fits, or rather immediately preceding them, he had always experienced a moment or two when his whole heart, and mind, and body seemed to wake up with vigor and light; when he became filled with joy and hope, and all his anxieties seemed to be swept away for ever; these moments were but presentiments, as it were, of the one final second ... in which the fit came upon him. That second, of course, was inexpressible. Next moment something appeared to burst open before him: a wonderful inner light illuminated his soul. This lasted perhaps half a second, yet he distinctly remembered hearing the beginning of a wail, the strange, dreadful wail, which burst from his lips of its own accord and which no effort of will on his part could suppress. Next moment he was absolutely unconscious; black darkness blotted out everything. He had fallen in an epileptic fit [7].

Temporal lobe epilepsy can be caused by a head injury or an infection which affects the brain. Most other causes are unknown [8].

Today, the seizures associated with temporal lobe epilepsy can be controlled very well by certain medications. These medications include dilantin, tegretol, trileptal, depakote, and frisium [8]. Treatment for temporal lobe epilepsy is considered to be more successful if combined with social rehabilitation at a young age [9].

Previously, individuals with temporal lobe epilepsy were treated by a surgical approach. Dr. Wilder Penfield, in the 1920's, was a pioneer in the development of the surgical approach to the treatment of epilepsy [10].

Modern medicine has used proton magnetic resonance spectroscopy in diagnosing temporal lobe epilepsy. This technique has proven useful in helping the treating medical professionals understand the underlying pathophysiology of temporal lobe epilepsy [11].

THE CONVERSION OF ST. PAUL AND TEMPORAL LOBE EPILEPSY

"I simply know that in the body or out of the body (God knows which) this man was caught up to paradise and heard sacred secrets which no human lips can repeat. Of an experience like that I am prepared to boast ... My wealth of visions might have puffed me up, so I was given a thorn in the flesh, an angel of Satan to rack me and keep me from being puffed up; three times over I prayed the Lord to relieve me of it, but he told me, "It is enough for you to have my grace: it is in weakness that my power is fully felt" [12]. These are the words of St. Paul describing some of his visions. Some would say these visions are induced by a medical condition while others argue that these visions are of a truly religious origin.

Nonetheless, the visions experienced by St. Paul started after he had set out from Jerusalem to Damascus with arrest warrants for certain early Christians [13]. Damascus is approximately 140 miles to the north of Jerusalem. En route Saul was knocked from his horse as a bright light flashed about him and a voice questioned him "Saul, Saul, why do you continue to persecute me?" [14]. He responded by asking, "Who are you?" The Bible states that the men with Saul were speechless at the response they heard but saw no one, "I am Jesus. I am the one you are so cruel to. Now get up and go into the city, where you will be told what to do." When Saul picked himself off the ground, he opened his eyes but was completely blind. For three days he was blind and did not eat or drink. Jesus then appeared to Ananias and said to him "Get up and go to the house of Judas on Straight Street. When you get there, you will find a man named Saul from the city of Tarsus. Saul is praying, and he has seen a vision. He saw a man named Ananias coming to him and putting his hands on him, so that he could see again." A reluctant Ananias found Saul and greeted him with the words, "Saul, the Lord Jesus has sent me. He is the same one who appeared to you along the road. He wants you to be able to see and to be filled with the Holy Spirit." [15] Saul was then baptized and the blind man could now see [13].

The conversion of St. Paul is a classic example of how the faithful attempt to explain the signs and symptoms of certain medical ailments as being the result of a divine intervention.

The events on the road to Damascus which were experienced by St. Paul can be attributed to a temporal lobe epileptic seizure- the voice, flash of light, blindness, loss of appetite (Table 7). However, it is wrong and foolish to dismiss the arguments of the faithful. The medical community certainly does not have all the answers. The true lesson to be learned from St. Paul's conversion experience is that science and religion have the same goal- to find out the truth- and to do such they must work together. Their motives and goals are more similar than either is usually willing to admit. The barrier is that although they both seek the same end, they speak two very different languages.

Table 7.   Signs and Symptoms of Temporal Lobe Epilepsy [6, 7]

-loss of normal body posture
-bright light
-hyperreligiosity
-hypergraphia
-hyposexuality
-epileptic seizures
-hallucinations
-an unawareness in the individual of having had a seizure
-sense of unprovoked fear

REFERENCES

[1]   Witherup RD. Introducing St. Paul the Apostle: his life and mission. Catholic Update July 2008; 1-4.

[2]   Acts 22: 3

[3]   New Advent. Gamaliel. Accessed on September 27, 2013. Available at: http://www.newadvent.org/cathen/06374b.htm

[4]   The Famous People. St. Paul Biography. Accessed on November 12, 2013. Available at: http://thefamouspeople.com/profiles/st-paul-91.php

[5]   Washington Times. Remains of St. Paul confirmed. June 29, 2009.

[6]   Epilepsy Foundation. Temporal Lobe Epilepsy. Accessed on 12/2/13. Available at: http://www.epilepsyfoundation.org/aboutepilepsy/syndromes/temporallobeepilepsy.cfm

[7]   Dostoyevsky F. The Idiot. Oxford University Press, 1988: 658 pages.

[8]   Epilepsy.com Temporal lobe epilepsy. Accessed on 12/23/13. Available at: http://www.epilepsy.com/epilepsy/epilepsy_temporallobe.epilepsy.com

[9]   Jensen I, Vaernet K. Temporal lobe epilepsy: follow-up investigation of 74 temporal lobe resected patients. Acta Neurochirurgica 37, 173-200 (1977).

[10] Rasmussen TB. Wilder Penfield: his legacy to neurology- surgical treatment of epilepsy. Can Med Assoc J 1977 June 18; 116(12)-1369-1370.

[11] Crass JH, Connelly A, Jackson GD, Johnson CL, Neville BG, Gadian DG. Proton magnetic resonance spectroscopy in children with temporal lobe epilepsy. Ann Neurol 1996 Jan; 39(1): 107-113.

[12] 2 Corinthians 12: 1-9

[13] Acts 9: 1ff

[14] Matthew 23: 37

[15] 1 Samuel 15: !

CHAPTER 24

The Habsburg Jaw

Abstract: The Habsburg jaw refers to the dominantly inherited trait which was present and clearly evident in the Habsburg family. This condition manifests itself as mandibular prognathism, jutting of the jaw and drooping of the lower lip. Charles II was the last Habsburg ruler of Spain. Charles II was physically and mentally disabled and died having produced no offspring. His death was followed by a chaotic period in which various factions struggled for political power.

Keywords: Abdominal pain, asthma, convulsions, diarrhea, drooping of lower lip, edema, genetics, Habsburg jaw, hallucinations, impotence, inbreeding, infertility, intermarriages, jutting of jaw.

CHARLES II OF SPAIN

The medical life of Charles II of Spain perfectly illustrates the devastating effects of inbreeding on the royal Habsburg family of Spain. Through the passage of time, the predominant clinical feature of this inbreeding has become known as the Habsburg jaw.

Charles II was born in November of 1661 in Madrid to Philip IV and his second wife (and niece), Maria. A nurse breast fed the feeble child until around the age of five. In an effort to not overburden the child, Charles was never educated and allowed to become extremely lazy in every aspect of his life.

Modern scientists have speculated that Charles' unique clinical characteristics were the result of combined pituitary hormone deficiency and distal renal tubular acidosis. Both of these disorders are genetic in origin. They can account for Charles' impotence and infertility [1].

Charles married twice- the first time at the age of 18 and the second time at 29. Both marriages produced no heirs. As an adult he suffered from hematuria, diarrhea, and edemas of his feet, abdomen, legs, and face. His health continued to decline in his 30's as he suffered from hallucinations and convulsions. His death at the age of 39 was preceded by fever, abdominal pain, difficulty breathing and coma [2].

Charles II died on November 1, 1700 but, his unique inbred physical characteristics will live on in his many royal portraits. One only needs to look at these portraits to be reminded of the devastating effects of inbreeding which led to the fall of the Spanish Habsburg dynasty (1516-1700).

THE HABSBURG JAW

Charles II is a well documented and obvious example of the condition which has become known as the Habsburg jaw. This term generally refers to the collective facial characteristics of the royal Habsburg family. These traits have been seen in nine generations of the family [3]. These traits include a prognathic mandible, a thick and everted lip, a large and misshapen nose with a prominent dorsal hump and an eversion of the lower eyelids. Systemic ailments include asthma, epilepsy, dropsy, gout, and melancholia [4, 5].

The physical facial deformities of the Habsburg family can be traced to the commonplace intermarriages between closely related individuals dating back to the thirteenth century. These traits have been expertly preserved for modern investigators in the many royal portraits of the various family members [4].

The hallmark of the Habsburg jaw is, predictably, the protrusion of the lower jaw. This is a result of the increased obtuseness of the angle between the body and ramus of the mandible [6]. This led to family members having difficulty swallowing, chewing, pronouncing certain words and even limiting the ability of certain family members to close their mouth. One family member was once told upon a visit to another country, "Your Majesty, shut your mouth, the flies of this country are very insolent."

The Habsburg dynasty ended with Charles II being brought down by their own consanguinous genetics.

REFERENCES

[1]   ABC Science. Inbreeding brought down Spanish dynasty. Accessed on December 31, 2013. Available at: http://www.abc.net.au/science/articles/2009/04/16/2544396.

[2]   Alvarez G, Ceballas FC, Quinteiro C. Recessive distal renal tubular acidosis and Charles II-an unlikely combination. Plosone; April 15, 2009. DOI: 10.1371/journal.pone.005174.

[3]   Grabb WC, Hodge GP, Dingman RO, O'Neal RM. The Habsburg jaw. Plast Reconst Surg 1958; 42: 442-445.

[4]   Hodge GP. A Medical history of the Spanish Habsburgs JAMA 1977 Sep 12; 238(11): 1169-1174.

[5]   Thompson EM and Winter RM. J Med Genet 1988 December; 25(12): 838-842.

[6]   Hart GD. The Habsburg jaw. Can Med Assoc J 1971 April 3; 104(7): 601-603.

CHAPTER 25

The Rapunzel Syndrome

Abstract: The Rapunzel syndrome is known in medical terminology as trichobezoar. It is a very rare disorder in which hair is swallowed by an individual. The hair is indigestable and becomes entrapped within the stomach resulting in a hair ball. After years of this condition the hairs start to extend beyond the stomach into the small bowel. This is known as the Rapunzel syndrome. It is primarily found in children who are emotionally disturbed. The syndrome takes its name from a Brothers Grimm's fairy tale character, Rapunzel. The fictional Rapunzel is known for her long, flowing, beautiful hair.

Keywords: Brothers Grimm, fairy tale, folktales, Hanau, laproscopy, Rapunzel syndrome, small bowel, stomach, trichobezoar, trichophagia, trichotillomania.

THE BROTHERS GRIMM

Philip Wilhelm Grimm was a lawyer and court official who lived in Hanau, Germany with his wife, Dorothea Grimm. The couple had nine children. On January 4, 1785 Jacob Ludwig Carl Grimm was born. A little over a year later Wilhelm Carl Grimm was born. Jacob and Wilhelm both studied law at the University of Marburg in the early 1800's. In 1808 Jacob and Wilhelm both took up positions as librarians at the Kassel School to support their younger siblings as both of their parents had passed away [1]. In 1812 they published a simple book of folktales which was followed up two years later by another volume containing 70 new stories. This book went on to become the best known book ever written in the German language [1].

The brothers eventually led an academic life. They were elected to the Berlin Academy of Sciences and went on to lecture for the remainder of their lives at Berlin University. Wilhelm died on December 16, 1859 and Jacob died on September 20, 1863 [2].

RAPUNZEL

Rapunzel is the main character in a Brothers Grimm's fairy tale [3]. The story starts with a childless couple who longs desperately for a child. The wife then becomes pregnant. During the pregnancy the husband made a deal with a sorceress to give the infant to her once the baby was born. When the wife gave birth the sorceress came and took the newborn and named her Rapunzel. Rapunzel grew into the most beautiful girl in the land.

When the little girl became twelve years-old the sorceress locked her away into a tower with no doors or stairway. It only had a tiny window at the top. The sorceress visited Rapunzel by making her unbraid her golden hair and letting it fall twenty yards to the ground so she could use the hair to climb up into the tower.

A prince was passing the tower and heard the beautiful Rapunzel singing. He did not know how to enter the tower because he saw no entrance. One day he saw the sorceress telling Rapunzel to let down her hair and climbed up the tower using Rapunzel's beautiful hair. She then climbed through the tower's small window. He thought he would try this himself. He finally met the beautiful Rapunzel and asked her to marry him. Rapunzel was delighted but she did not know how she could escape the tower. They decided that he would visit her every night bringing a strand of silk which she would weave together to escape.

The wicked sorceress found out about their plan and was furious. She took Rapunzel into the woods and cut off her beautiful hair. She then took the hair back to the tower and lowered it down to the unsuspecting prince. The prince was greeted in the tower by the evil and hideous woman rather than the beautiful Rapunzel.

The grief stricken prince threw himself out of the tower into a bed of thorns which blinded him. The prince then wandered the forest for years before coming upon Rapunzel. Rapunzel recognized him and threw her arms around him. Two of Rapunzel's tears fell into the prince's eyes bringing back his sight. They then went off to the prince's kingdom to live happily together.

The fairy tale of Rapunzel has been popular with children worldwide through the years and has been subjected to many popular references. In 2010 Disney released an animated movie, 'Tangled', featuring the enchanted long-haired beauty [4].

THE RAPUNZEL SYNDROME

The Rapunzel syndrome is a rare form of trichobezoar. It is found in a very limited number of individuals who have psychiatric disorders, trichotillomania (the habit of hair pulling) and trichophagia (the habit of chewing hair) (Table **8**). This rare combination of habits results in the development of gastric bezoars [5]. This syndrome was first reported in the literature in 1968 [6] and takes its name from the Grimm Brothers' fictional young girl with long flowing hair. This syndrome is characterized by a long tail extending beyond the duodenum.

Table 8.   Signs and Symptoms of Rapunzel Syndrome [7, 8]

-palpable abdominal mass
-weakness
-weight loss
-constipation
-diarrhea
-nausea
-low hemoglobin levels
-vomiting

The diagnostic procedure for Rapunzel syndrome is endoscopy. A CT scan is useful to see the extension of the trichobezoar [7]. Small trichobezoars may be resolved by endoscopic removal [7, 8]. Laproscopy and a laser ignited mini-explosive technique have also been used with success [7, 9]. However, open surgery is the most reliable treatment method for large trichobezoars which have extended into the bowel.

The proper treatment of Rapunzel syndrome consists of early diagnosis, removal of the bezoar, and re-evaluation appointments [10]. Selective serotonin reuptake inhibitors have been recommended in the treatment of the trichotillomania aspect of the syndrome [11]. Behavioral therapy is recommended to control the trichophagia [11, 12].

REFERENCES

[1]   Ashliman D.L. Grimm Brothers' home page. Accessed on October 11, 2013. Available at: http://www.pitt.edu/-dash/grimm.html#chronology.

[2]   World of tales. The Brothers Grimm biography. Accessed on October 11, 2013. Available at: http://www.worldoftales.com/fairy_tales/Brothers_Grimm_biography.html

[3]   Jacob and Wilhelm Grimm, "Rapunzel," Kinder-und Hausmarchen, gesammelt durch die Bruder Grimm [Children's and Household Tales-Grimms' Rairy Tales], 7th ed., vol. 1 (Gottingen: Verlag der Dieterichschen Buchhandlung, 1857), no. 12, pp. 65-69.

[4]   Imdb. Tangled. Accessed on October 11, 2013. Available at: http://www.imdb.com/title/tt0398286/.

[5]   Lopes LR, Oliveira PSP, Pracucho EM, Camargo MA, de Souza Coelho Neto J, Andreollo NA. The Rapunzel dyndrome: an unusual trichobezoar presentation. Case Reports in medicine Volume 2010 (2010) article ID 841028, 3 pages.

[6]   Vaughan ED, Sawyers JL, Scott HW. The Rapunzel syndrome: an unusual complication of intestinal bezoar. Surgery 1968; vol 63, (2): 339-343.

[7]   Al Wadan AH, Al Kaff H, Al Senabani J, Al Saad AA. 'Rapunzel syndrome' trichobezoa in a 7-year-old girl: a case report. Cases Journal 2008; 1: 205.

[8]   Gupta Naik S, Naik S, Chaudhary AK, Jain P, Sharma A: Rapunzel Syndrome Reviewed and Redefined. Dig Surg 2007, 24: 157-161.

[9]   Dumonceaux A, Michaud L, Bonnevalle M, Debeugny P, Gottard F, Turk D: Trichobezoar in children and adolescent. Arch Paediatr 1998, 5: 996-999.

[10]   Huang YC, Liu QS, Guo ZH: The use of laser ignited mini-explosive technique in treating 100 cases of gastric bezoars. Chung Hua Nei Ko Tsa chih 1994, 33: 172-174.

[11]   Middleton E, Macksey LF, Phillips JD. Rapunzel syndrome in a pediatric patient: a case report. AANA Journal April 2012; 80(2): 115-119.

[12]   Gonuguntla V, Joshi D. Rapunzel syndrome: a 'comprehensive review of an unusual case of a trichobezoar. Clin Med Res 2009; 7(3): 99-102.

CHAPTER 26

The Peter Pan Syndrome

Abstract: As a child, James M. Barrie was deeply affected by the death of his thirteen year-old older brother. Barrie developed into a very successful and celebrated author. In 1904, Peter Pan first appeared as a play and, subsequently, as a novel seven years later. Barrie celebrated the freedom and joys of childhood in his masterpiece. Peter Pan Syndrome refers to individuals, mainly males, who have experienced an abnormal psychological halt to the maturation process of their personality traits. These individuals lack self-confidence, avoid long-term relationships, cannot make commitments, and usually do not honor their promises.

Keywords: Llewelyn-Davies boys, manipulative, Peter Pan, pneumonia, self-confidence, self-pity, Tiger Lily, undependable.

J.M. BARRIE

James Barrie was born to Scottish weavers on May 9, 1860 in Kirriemuir, Forfarshire, Scotland [1]. For the first six years of his life, and in essence for his entire childhood, Barrie was overshadowed in his family by his older brother, David, who was the focus of their mother's love and attention.

On the day before David's fourteenth birthday, in January of 1867, David was killed in a skating accident. Their mother was inconsolable and never mentally recovered from this tragedy [2].

His mother's sorrow over the loss of David and future conversations with her shaped Barrie's thoughts and, in turn, his writings. He would believe, as an adult, that there was nothing worthwhile that could occur in a male's life after the age of twelve. He later wrote, 'She lived twenty-nine years after his death ... But I had not made her forget the bit of her that was dead; in those nine-and twenty years he was not removed one day farther from her. Many a time she fell asleep speaking to him, and even while she slept her lips moved and she smiled as if he had come back to her, and when she woke he might vanish so suddenly that she started up bewildered and looked about her, and then said slowly, "My David's dead!" or perhaps he remained long enough to whisper why he must leave her now, and then she lay silent with filmy eyes. When I became a man ... he was still a boy of thirteen."

Barrie graduated from Edinburgh University in 1882. He began writing popular novels such as 'A Window in Thrums' (1889) and moved to London. While living in London he took long walks through Kensington Gardens where, in the late 1890's, he met the five Llewelyn-Davies brothers. Barrie would eventually become their guardian after the death of their parents. His relationship with these boys served as the inspiration for his masterpiece- Peter Pan [1].

Barrie went on to write prodigiously for the rest of his life and to receive many accolades. He was awarded, in 1913, the Knight Bachelor of the Order of the British Empire.

The five Llewelyn-Davies boys could not escape the realities of life. Life for them certainly was not a fantastical existence in Neverland. Michael drowned in 1921, George was killed in military service in 1915 and Peter committed suicide in 1960. Barrie himself passed away on June 19, 1937 of pneumonia [3].

Barrie's admiration and love of the childhood state of being has had a profound tangible effect on the well-being of thousands of British youths through the decades. In 1929 Barrie gave all the rights to Peter Pan to a London children's hospital- The Great Ormond Street Hospital. The Hospital was stunned when he gave his rights to them. The British Parliament gave an exemption to the Hospital in 2007 as the copyright term was set to expire. Great Ormond Street Hospital, because of this exemption, is able to help children with the royalties from Peter Pan in perpetuity [4].

PETER PAN OR THE BOY WHO WOULDN'T GROW UP

'All children, except one, grow up. They soon know that they will grow up and the way Wendy knew was this. One day when she was two years old she was playing in a garden and she plucked another flower and ran with it to her mother. I suppose she must have looked rather delightful' for Mrs. Darling put her hand to her heart and cried, 'Oh, why can't you remain like this forever!'" This was all that passed between them on the subject, but henceforth Wendy knew that she must grow up. You always know after you are two. Two is the beginning of the end [5]'.

Such is how the adventures of Peter Pan begin. In so doing it offers the reader a glimpse into the soul of Barrie.

Peter Pan was released, in 1904, in the form of a play and, in 1911, as a novel. It delighted countless children of all nations for generations. It has been the subject of numerous movies, television shows, Broadway and London theatrical productions, documentaries, and analytical essays. It has given the world the immortal characters of Peter Pan, Wendy Darling, Tinker Bell, the Lost Boys, Tiger Lily, and Captain Hook.

The general theme of the book is that the most desirable thing to be possessed would be never ending youth- a youth filled with adventure, freedom, and a carefree environment free from the grotesque intrusions of the real world.

PETER PAN SYNDROME

The Peter Pan Syndrome is a term coined by Dr. Dan Kiley [6]. It refers to individuals, particularly men, who act in an immature manner.

Individuals with the Peter Pan Syndrome are characterized by a lack of self confidence, an inability to take constructive criticism, and an inability to make commitments or to keep promises (Table **9**). Also, they are usually always looking for a younger partner [7] in an effort to avoid stressful situations which might necessitate making plans for the future.

Table 9.   Signs and Symptoms of Peter Pan Syndrome [8]

-wrathful anger
-self pity
-difficulty expressing emotions
-depression
-undependable
-manipulative
-happiness that turns to panic

REFERENCES

[1]   Bio.true story. J.M. Barrie biography. Accessed on September 29, 2013, Available at: http://www.bio.com/people/jm_barrie_9200058.

[2]   Birkin A. J.M. Barrie and the lost boys: the real story. Yale University Press; New Haven and London: 2003.

[3]   Imdb. JM. Barrie. Accessed on: September 30, 2013. Available at: http://www.imdb.com/name/nm0057381/bio.

[4]   Allen K. Never ends for Peter Pan. The Guardian. December 28, 2007.

[5]   Barrie J.M. Peter and Wendy. October 1911. Charles Scribner's Sons.

[6]   Kiley D. The Peter Pan Syndrome: men who have never grown up. Corgi Books. October 26, 1984.

[7]   Science News. Overprotective parents can lead children to develop 'Peter Pan Syndrome.' Accessed on October 1, 2013. Available at: http://www.sciencedaily.com/releases/2007/05/070501112023.htm

[8]   SyndromesPedia. What are the symptoms of Peter Pan Syndrome? Accessed on 9/30/13. Available at: syndromespedia.com/peter-pan-syndrome.html.

CHAPTER 27

Damien the Leper

Abstract: Pope Benedict XVI canonized Father Damien de Veuster on October 11, 2009. Dr. Damien commenced his ministry, in 1873, in which he would serve those individuals who were afflicted with leprosy and quarantined in Molokai on the Hawaiian Islands. He eventually contracted the disease and died of it in 1889. Leprosy is a disease which is caused by *Mycobacterium leprae*. It has a long incubation period and is not very contagious. Presently the disease is treated with antibiotics and the patient can live a normal life if the disease is diagnosed at an early stage.

Keywords: Cholera, clofazimine, Congregation of the Fathers of the Sacred Hearts of Jesus and Mary, Damien, dapsone, Hansen's disease, influenza, leprosy, Molokai, *Mycobacterium leprae*, rifampin, smallpox, tuberculosis, venereal disease.

ST. DAMIEN OF MOLOKAI

Josef De Veuster was born on January 3, 1884 in Tremelo, Belgium. He entered, at the age of 19, the Congregation of the Fathers of the Sacred Hearts of Jesus and Mary [1]. Here, he would take the religious name of Damien. During his novitiate at the Congregation, Damien would pray every day before a picture of the patron saint of missionaries, St. Francis Xavier. Damien longed for his superiors to send him on a mission [2].

Damien had a brother, Pamphile, who was a priest in the same congregation as Damien. Pamphile was assigned to the Hawaiian Islands but, fell very ill and was not able to travel. Damien volunteered to fill his brother's position. He arrived in Hawaii in March of 1864 and was ordained a priest in Honolulu two months later [3].

In the 1700's the first European explorers, under the command of Captain Cook, reached the Hawaiian Islands. These Europeans were greeted in this Pacific paradise by approximately 300,000 native inhabitants. By the late 1800's the Hawaiian population shrunk to 50,000. Through the years smallpox, venereal disease, cholera, influenza, tuberculosis, and leprosy were introduced to the native population.

Leprosy, like no other disease, struck terror into the hearts of all that came into contact with it. For thousands of years government officials throughout the world dealt with the deadly disease by isolating the afflicted from the general community. Hawaiian officials were no different. The Hawaiian government set up a leper colony on the island of Molokai in 1868 [4].

Upon arrival at the leper settlement, lepers were told by the ship's sailors to jump overboard and swim to shore. Occasional supplies would be thrown into the water and the current would hopefully wash them ashore to the exiles.

Fr. Damien arrived at Kalaupapa in 1873. He provided for the inhabitants spiritual needs, built homes, churches, and coffins, and advocated the government in Honolulu to provide better medical services and funding [5]. He freely gave of his physical body and willingly made himself a leper.

In 1884 it was announced that Fr. Damien had contracted the dreaded disease. At the age of 49, Fr. Damien died on April 15, 1889. He was buried under a Pandanus tree. It was the same spot where he had first slept upon his arrival to the cursed isle sixteen years prior [7].

Today, the heroic sacrifices of the Belgian priest are celebrated worldwide. On October 11, 2009 Damien of Molokai was canonized a saint by the Roman Catholic Church. His canonization was attended by Belgium's King Albert and Queen Paola [6]. The President of the United States, Barack Obama, who grew up in Hawaii, sent a message which read, in part, "In our own time as millions around the world suffer from disease, especially the pandemic of HIV/AIDS, we should draw on the example of Fr. Damien's resolve in answering the urgent call to heal and care for the sick."

There is also a beautiful, yet simple, bronze statue of Damien in the rotunda of the United States Capitol Building. It clearly shows the effects of the dreaded disease on Damien's body.

During Damien's canonization homily, Pope Benedict XVI said "Let us remember before this noble figure that it is charity which makes unity, brings it forth and makes it desirable. Following in St. Paul's footsteps, St. Damien prompts us to choose the good warfare, not the kind that brings division but the kind that gathers people together. He invites us to open our eyes to the forms of leprosy that disfigure the humanity of our brethren and still today call for the charity of our presence as servants, beyond that of our generosity."

LEPROSY

An acid-fast, rod-shaped bacillus known as *Mycobacterium leprae* is the cause of leprosy. It is a chronic disease which causes disfigurement and physical disabilities that affects the skin, eyes, peripheral nerves and the mucosa of the upper respiratory tract [8]. Leprosy, also known as Hansen's disease, has a very long incubation period and is not very contagious. Almost 95% of the population worldwide has a natural immunity to leprosy [9]. Children are more susceptible than adults to the disease [10].

The mode of transmission of leprosy is still not very well understood. However, it is known that prolonged contact with a person who has the disease is required for one to catch it.

There are two forms of leprosy. They are tuberculoid and lepromatous. Tuberculoid leprosy has few skin lesions while there are many skin lesions in lepromatous leprosy [10]. The signs and symptoms of leprosy include muscle weakness, skin lesions and numbness in hands, arms, feet, and legs.

Antibiotics are used to treat leprosy. Theses antibiotics include rifampin, clofazimine, and dapsone [9]. Once an individual is placed on medications he or she becomes noninfectious. Ergo, it is imperative that contact be avoided with untreated individuals as a form of prevention [11-13].

REFERENCES

[1]   Living with Christ Staff. St. Damien Joseph de Veuster. Accessed on October 23, 2013. Available at: http://www.catholicdigest.com/articles/faith/saints/2011/05-08/st- damien-joseph-de-veuster

[2]   Vatican, St. Jozef Damien De Veuster (1840-1889). Accessed on October 12, 2013. Available at: http://www.vatican.va/news_services/liturgy/saints/2009/ ns_lit_doc_200910 11_de_veuster_en.htnl.

[3]   American Catholic.org. St. Damien Joseph de Veuster of Moloka'i. Accessed on October 30, 2013. Available at: http://www.americancatholic.org/features/saints/ saint.aspx?id=1 379.

[4]   Global Catholic Network. St. Damien of Molokai. Accesses on October 21, 2013. Available at: www.ewtn.com/saintsholy/saints/D/stdamienofmolokai.asp.

[5]   Visitmoloki.com. Moloka'i Kalaupapa. Accessed on October 24, 2013. Available at: http://visitmolokai.com/kala.html.

[6]   Stewart R. Leper Priest of Molokai: the Father Damien Story. July 2000; University of Hawai'i Press; 452 pp.

[7]   Architect of the Capitol. Damien. Accessed on: October 31, 2013. Available at: http://www.aoc.gov/capitol-hill/national-statuary-hill-collection/father-damien.

[8]   World Health Organization. Leprosy: the disease. Accessed on September 29, 2013. Available at: http:www.who.int/lep/leprosy/en/index.html.

[9]   American Leprosy Missions. Leprosy Frequently Asked Questions. Accessed on October 20, 2013. Available at: http://www.leprosy.org/leprosy_faqs.

[10]   New York State Government. Leprosy (Hansen's disease). Accessed on 10/31/13. Available at: http://www.health.ny.gov/diseases/communicable/leprosy/fact_sheet.htm.

[11]   MedlinePlus. leprosy. Accessed on October 31, 2013. Available at: http:// www.nih.gov/medlineplus/ency/article/001347.

[12]   Renault CA, Ernst JD. *Mycobacterium leprae*. In: Mandell GL, Bennett JE, Dolin R, eds. Principles and Practice of Infectious Diseases. 7th ed. Philadelphia, Pa: Elsevier Churchill Livingstone; 2009: chap 251.

[13]   Ernst JD. Leprosy (Hansen's disease). In: Goldman L, Ausiello D, eds. Cecil Medicine. 24th ed. Philadelphia, Pa: Saunders Elsevier; 2011: chap 334.

CHAPTER 28

Louis Braille's Gift to the Visually Impaired

Abstract: Louis Braille was born in France in the early 1800's. Braille suffered an accident in his father's workshop which severely damaged one of his eyes. An infection ensued and spread to the other eye causing the child to become completely blind by the age of five. As a young man, Braille developed a system of reading and writing for the blind and visually impaired. He based his system on a highly imperfect system of night reading developed by the French military. Today Braille's system is accepted and implemented worldwide.

Keywords: Accidents, contracted braille, diabetes, diagnosis, French military, glaucoma, intraocular pressure, macular degeneration, optic disc cupping, systemic disease, uncontracted braille, vision.

LOUIS BRAILLE

Louis Braille was born on January 4, 1809 in Coupvray, France. Coupvray is a small town near Paris. Braille was very fond of physical work when he was a very young child. One day he was working in his father's harness workshop. He began working on a piece of leather with an awl. The tool slid and punctured his eye. The damaged eye became infected and soon spread to his other eye. At the age of three Louis Braille was blind in both eyes [1].

Louis was an intelligent child and, when he was ten years old, he was awarded a scholarship to the Institut National des Jeunes Aveugles in Paris. This was the first school in the world designed exclusively for the education of blind children. This scholarship was not only fortuitous for young Louis but, would prove to be a gift for the visually impaired for years to come.

Two years after entering the school a former soldier named Charles Barbier was invited to speak to the students [2]. Charles Barbier was born in Valenciennes on May 18, 1767. Barbier's father was comptroller of the King's Farms and arranged for him to enter a military academy at the age of 15. He graduated as an artillery officer and emigrated to America where he worked as a land surveyor. He soon developed a keen interest in codes and developed a system of reading which he referred to as 'night writing'. The primary purpose of 'night writing' was to allow military officers to read and write at night without having their location detected.

Upon learning of Barbier's system, 12 year old Louis Braille became very enthused and wished to make suggestions to Barbier to improve his system. However, Barbier was not interested in receiving any suggestions from Louis and eventually took an interest in the deaf-and-dumb [3].

Louis went on to simplify Barbier's system and developed a system of his own based on normal spelling which used six dots to represent the standard alphabet. Braille became a respected teacher at the Institute but his system was not widely used during his lifetime.

Louis died of tuberculosis on January 6, 1852. His body was exhumed by the French government one hundred years later, in 1952, to be reburied in the Pantheon in Paris with other French national heroes [4].

VISUAL IMPAIRMENT

Visual impairment affects, to varying degrees, millions of individuals worldwide. Causes of visual impairment include various pathologies, age, accidents, and systemic diseases such as diabetes. In France alone there are 3,346,000 individuals representing various age groups which have some form of visual impairment [5]. In the United States, individuals with vision worse than 20/200 with glasses or contact lenses are considered to be legally blind [6].

The leading cause of loss of vision in individuals over 65 years of age is age-related macular degeneration (AMD). Another leading cause of vision loss in the aged population is glaucoma. Primary open-angle glaucoma is the most prevalent form of glaucoma. It is a chronic, slowly progressive disorder which is characterized by increased optic disc cupping, visual field loss, open and normal-appearing angles, and intraocular pressure greater than 21 mm Hg.

In order to prevent or forestall increased vision loss it is imperative that there is early detection, diagnosis, and treatment [7]. Early detection can lead to corrective measures for one's vision and, in some cases, a diagnosis of a previously undetected systemic disorder.

BRAILLE

The work of young Louis Braille benefits millions of visually impaired individuals worldwide. This system allows the individual to both read and write through touch. In the braille system each letter in the alphabet is represented by a unique dot configuration. The ability to name individual characters is one of the earliest braille literacy skills [8]. Producing and combining letter sounds are more complex braille-reading skills which can only be learned after the basic skills are mastered [9]. Some people think that braille is a language. This is a misconception. Braille is not a language but a code by which any language may be read or written. Braille cells are units of space in which braille symbols are formed. A full braille cell is made up of six raised dots. These six raised dots are arranged in two parallel rows. Each of these two parallel rows has three dots. Using these dots, there are 64 possible combinations. Each cell can represent a punctuation mark, number, whole word, or alphabet letter [10]. Experienced braille readers can read braille at a rate of 200 to 400 words per minute [11].

There are two grades of braille. They are uncontracted braille and contracted braille. Uncontracted braille is a straightforward letter for letter translation from print. Contracted braille can decrease the size of braille documents by approximately 25% as it has special signs for combinations of letters and common words [12]. Much academic research has led to improvements in the way braille is taught and understood. One group of researchers recently created a computerized program to teach visual braille reading. This might have tremendous future implications [13].

REFERENCES

[1]   American Foundation for the Blind. Louis Braille Biography. Accessed on October 9, 2013. Available at: http://braillebug.afb/louis_braille_bio_asp.

[2]   NNDB. Louis Braille. Accessed on November 27, 2013. Available at: http://www.nndb.com/people/971/000086713/.

[3]   The Valentin Hauy Association. Biographies. Accessed on November 27, 2013. Available at: http://www.avh.asso.fr/Rubrics/association/biographies.php?langue=eng.

[4]   CNIB. Biography of Louis Braille.Accessed on November 27, 2013. Available at: http://www.cnib.ca/en/living/braille/louis-braille-/Pages/default.aspx.

[5]   OPC Association. Visual Impairment. Accessed on November 26, 2013. Available at: http://www.opc.asso.fr/?Visual-Impairment+lang=en&gclid=cPzyu_eOhbsCFbB90godn68 AKA.

[6]   Quillen DA. Common causes of vision loss in elderly patients. Am Fam Physician. 1999 Jul 1; 60(1): 99-108.

[7]   Scripps. Discover blindness. Accessed on November 27, 2013. Available at: http://www.scripps.edu/discover/blindness.html.

[8]   Toussaint KA, Tiger JH. Teaching early braille literacy skills within a stimulus equivalence paradigm to children with degenerative visual impairments. J Appl Behav Anal 2010 Summer; 43(2): 181-194.

[9]   Hampshire BE. Tactile and visual reading. New Outlook for the Blind 1975; 69: 145-154.

[10]   American Foundation for the Blind. What is Braille? Accessed on October 22, 2013. Available at: http://www.afb.org/section.aspx?FolderID=2&SectionID=6&TopicID=199.

[11]   National Federation of the Blind. Braille- what is it? Future Reflections 1996; 15(1).

[12]   RNIB. Six little dots. Accessed on October 22, 2013. Available at: http://www.rnib.org.uk/livingwithsightloss/reading/how/braille/braille/Pages/ what_is_braille.aspx.

[13]   Scheithauer MC, Tiger JH, Miller SJ. On the efficacy of a computer based program to teach visual braille reading. J Appl Behav Anal 2013 Jan; 46(2): 436-443.

CHAPTER 29

The Cocaine Addiction of Sir Arthur Conan Doyle's Sherlock Holmes

Abstract: The brilliant British detective, Sherlock Holmes, has fascinated millions worldwide with his uncanny ability to solve crimes by using the most miniscule of clues. The reader learns much about this character- a creation of the mind of Sir Arthur Conan Doyle. One of the darker characteristics of Sherlock Holmes is his cocaine addiction. The personality and thought processes of the fictional character are very similar to those of many real-life ordinary individuals. They think that they can use cocaine when life is not very exciting and avoid it during other more stimulating periods. This erroneous thought process can lead to many horrible complications and manifestations of cocaine use. Not least among these complications is addiction.

Keywords: Bruxism, Cocaine, dopamine, headaches, lidocaine, occlusal wear, photograph, spiritualism, tooth decay.

SIR ARTHUR CONAN DOYLE

On May 22, 1859 Charles Altamont Doyle and his wife, Mary (Foley) Doyle, welcomed their son, Arthur Ignatius Conan Doyle, into the world. The birth of the future 'father of the detective story' occurred in Edinburgh, Scotland. The family was a fairly prosperous Irish-Catholic family but, Arthur's father was an alcoholic.

When Arthur was nine years-old he was sent to England for schooling much to his displeasure. There were brutal physical punishments at Arthur's Jesuit school. This was the norm for the time in English schools [1].

Arthur later studied medicine and graduated from Edinburgh University in 1885 and practiced medicine until 1891 when he decided to devote all his time to his writing. Doyle's time studying medicine at Edinburgh University influenced the development of his most famous literary character, Sherlock Holmes. Sherlock

Holmes was based primarily on Dr. Joseph Bell. Dr. Bell was a surgeon and a member of the faculty. He amazed students with his unique ability to diagnose patients' ailments. The character development of Sherlock Holmes was also influenced by a teacher of forensic medicine, Sir Henry Littlejohn [2]. Sherlock Holmes received his name from a combination of a prominent violinist, Alfred Sherlock, and the American jurist, Oliver Wendell Holmes. Sherlock Holmes' partner received his moniker from Dr. John Watson who was a Southsea doctor and Portsmouth Literary and Scientific Society member [2].

The Sherlock Holmes stories have become immensely popular worldwide inspiring many references in the popular culture. The Sherlock Holmes canon consists of four novels and 56 short stories [3].

Later in life Doyle became deeply involved in spiritualism after his son died in World War I [4]. Sir Arthur Conan Doyle was absolutely confident that spirits exist. He would offer as proof of the existence of spirits Doyle offered a photograph of himself with the face of his dead son looking over his shoulder. Doyle insisted that he had developed the photograph himself and that nobody else ever touched it.

Upon Doyle's death on July 7, 1930 the writer's surviving son, Adrian Conan Doyle, stated "Why, of course, my father fully believed that when he passed over he would continue to keep in touch with us. All his family believe so, too ... There is no question that my father will often speak to us, just as he did before he passed over. We will always know when he is speaking, but one has to be careful because there are practical jokers on the other side, as there are here ... It is quite possible that these jokers may attempt to impersonate him. But there are tests which my mother knows, such as little mannerisms of speech which cannot be impersonated and which will tell us it is my father himself who is speaking [5]."

COCAINE

Cocaine is a very popular illicit drug used in nations throughout the world. Cocaine (benzoylmethlecgonine) is an alkaloid which is extracted from the leaf of the erythroxylon coca bush [6]. Peru and Bolivia are the primary locations where coca bushes are grown while they are refined primarily in Columbia [6, 8]. Drug dealers mix it with other substances in order to increase the quantity of their product. This has resulted in an extremely dangerous and potentially fatal side effect of the user not knowing how much cocaine is actually being ingested [8].

Cocaine is classified as a psychostimulant which exhibits both local anesthetic and neurotransmitter effects [9-12]. Centrally, cocaine affects adrenergic nerve endings which block the re-uptake of catecholamines and potentiates [13] particularly dopamine. This results in cocaine's transient euphoric effects [13, 14]. Locally, cocaine blocks the initiation and propagation of nerve impulses along an axon by interference with sodium permeability during depolarization [7, 14, 15].

There are many dental effects [6, 9, 16-21] of cocaine use which both the cocaine user and his/her dentist must be aware of and take into consideration when trying to determine the cause of a particular dental/oral condition and in possibly making modifications to usual treatment. They are: gingival lesions, tempromandibular disorders, bruxism, cervical abrasion, occlusal wear, corrosion of gold dental restorations, excessive hemorrhage after tooth extraction, increased rate of tooth decay, and increased rate of periodontal disease. Other intra-oral and craniofacial manifestations [6, 9, 17-23] include oral candidal infections, nasal necrosis, headaches, perforation of palate, oral ulcers, bilateral cleft lip and palate in fetus, xerostomia, angular cheilitis, halitosis, glossodynia, and erosive lichen planus. The administration of a local anesthetic with vasoconstrictor may result in an acute rise in blood pressure [6, 21]. There is also a risk of convulsions associated with the combination of lidocaine and cocaine potentiates [6, 24-27]. Use of epinephrine-impregnated retraction cords is also contraindicated [17]. All dental treatment should be postponed for at least 6 to 24 hours after the use of cocaine [6, 24, 27-30].

THE COCAINE USE OF SHERLOCK HOLMES

"Sherlock Holmes took his bottle from the corner of the mantel-piece and his hypodermic syringe from its neat morocco case. With his long, white, nervous fingers he adjusted the delicate needle, and rolled back his left shirt-cuff. For some little time his eyes rested thoughtfully upon the sinewy forearm and wrist all dotted and scarred with innumerable puncture-marks. Finally he thrust the sharp point home, pressed down the tiny piston, and sank back into the velvet-lined arm-chair with a long sigh of satisfaction [31]." These are the startling words which are found in the Sherlock Holmes story 'Sign of Four' [31] (Table **10**).

Table 10.   Possible Dental/Craniofacial Manifestations of Cocaine Use [34-55]

• TMD
• Bruxism
• Cervical abrasion
• Occlusal wear
• Corrosion of gold dental restorations
• Excessive hemorrhage after tooth extraction
• Increased rate of tooth decay
• Increased rate of periodontal disease
• Oral candidal infections
• Nasal necrosis
• Headaches
• Perforation of palate
• Oral ulcers
• Bilateral cleft lip and palate in fetus
• Xerostomia
• Angular cheilitis
• Halitosis
• Glossdynia
• Erosive lichen planus

The cocaine use of Sherlock Holmes has long been analyzed by scholars. They have asked why Sir Arthur Conan Doyle would make cocaine use an integral aspect of the persona of Sherlock Holmes. Holmes' cocaine use has even been compared to that of another brilliant investigator, Sigmund Freud [32]. There seems to be a connection between the two- at least in the mind of Arthur Conan Doyle.

Sigmund Freud wrote a paper entitled 'Uber Coca' which is believed to be Arthur Conan Doyle's inspiration for making cocaine addiction a part of the Sherlock Holmes persona. Freud became interested in the effects of cocaine after learning of Bavarian soldiers who were given cocaine in order to increase their battlefield endurance [33] (Table **11**).

Table 11. Informal Terms Referring to Cocaine [34]

-	Coke
-	Charlie
-	Snow
-	Flake
-	Blow
-	Toot
-	Aunt
-	Uptown
-	Yao
-	Dream
-	Foo-foo dust
-	White dragon

Whatever the true inspiration was, the true lesson to be learned from Sherlock Holmes is the potential for addiction of individuals of every socio-economic class and the shackling powers of cocaine addiction.

Extremely little was known about the effects of cocaine and addiction, in general, during the lifetime of Sir Arthur Conan Doyle. Today, we know of the litany of deleterious systemic effects of this illicit drug. Some individuals think, erroneously, like Sherlock Holmes, that they can add an excitement to their own lives through a recreational use of cocaine and then cease its use when they have more interesting and stimulating tasks at hand. This is a very dangerous thought process and usually ends by placing the user on the lost highway of addiction.

REFERENCES

[1]   Sir Arthur Conan Doyle Literary Estate. Sir Arthur Conan Doyle Biography. Accessed on 10/21/13. Available at: http:www.sherlockholmesonline.org/Biography/index.htm.

[2]   The Sherlock Holmes Society of London. Sir Arthur Conan Doyle. Accessed on 10/21/13. Available at: http://www.sherlock_holmes.org.uk/world/conan_doyle.php.

[3]   The Telegraph. October 21, 2013. Sir Arthur Conan Doyle's Sherlock Holmes in a case of identity.

[4]   Ross D. Sir Arthur Conan Doyle Biography. Accessed on October 21, 2013. Available at: http://www.britainexpress.com/History/bio/doyle.htm.

[5]   The New York Times. July 7, 1930. Conan Doyle dead from heart attack.

[6]   Brand HS, Gonggrijp S, Blanksma CJ. Cocaine and oral health. British Dental Journal 2008; 204: 365-369.

[7]   Children's Hospital of Philadelphia. Cocaine toxicity, Part I 2009; available at: www.chop.edu/consumer/jsp/division/generic.jsp?id=72612.

[8]   Cleveland Clinic. Cocaine and crack 2009; Available at: http://my.clevelandclinic.org/drugs/cocaine_crack/hic_cocaine_and_crack.aspx.

[9]   Villa PD. Midfacial complications of prolonged cocaine snort. J Can Dent Assoc 1999; 65: 218-223.

[10]   Goldstein FJ. Toxicity of cocaine. Compendium 1990; 11: 710, 712, 714-716.

[11]   Sastry RC, Lee D, Har-El G. Palatal perforation from cocaine abuse. Otolaryngol Head Neck Surg 1997; 116: 565-566.

[12]   Schweitzer V. Osteolytic sinusitis and pneumomediastinum: deceptive otolaryngologic complications of cocaine abuse. Laryngoscope 1986; 96: 206-210.

[13]   Bains MK, Hosseini-Ardehali M. Palatal perforations: past and present. Two case reports and a literature review. British Dental Journal 2005; 199: 267-269.

[14]   Lancaster J, Belloso A, Wison CA, McCormick M. Rare case of naso-oral fistula with extensive osteocartilaginous necrosis secondary to cocaine abuse: review of otorhinolaryngological presentations in cocaine addicts. J Laryngol Otol 2000; 114: 630-633.

[15]   Cregler LL, Mark H. Medical complications of cocaine abuse. N Engl J Med 1986 Dec 4; 315(23): 1495-1500.

[16]   Gay GR. Clinical management of acute and chronic cocaine poisoning. Ann Emerg Med 1982 Oct; 11(10): 562-572.

[17]   Blanksma CJ, Brand HS. Cocaine abuse: orofacial manifestations and implications for dental treatment. Int Dent J 2005; 55(6): 365-369.

[18]   Parry J, Porter S, Scully C, Flint S, Parry MG. Mucosal lesions due to oral cocaine use. Br Dent J 1996; 180; 462-464.

[19]   Brown RS, Johnson CD. Corrosion of gold restorations from inhalation of "crack" cocaine. Gen Dent 1994; 242-246.

[20]   Johnson CD, Brown RS. How cocaine abuse affects post-extraction bleeding. JADA 1993; 124: 60-62.

[21]   Mitchell-Lewis DA, Phelan JA, Kelly RB, Bradley JJ Lamster IB. Identifying oral lesions associated with crack cocaine use. J Am Dent Assoc 1994; 125(8): 1104-1108.

[22]   Mattson-Gates G, Jabs AD, Hugo NE. Perforation of the hard palate associated with cocaine abuse. Ann Plast Surg 1991; 29: 466-468.

[23]   Goodger NM, Wang J, Pogrel MA. Palatal and nasal necrosis resulting from cocaine misuse. Br Dent J 2005; 198: 333-334.

[24]   Yagiela JA. Adverse drug interactions in dental practice: interactions associated with vasoconstrictors. Part V of a series. J Am Dent Assoc 1999; 130: 701-709.

[25]   Engel JD. Cocaine: a historical and modern perspective. Nebr Med J 1991; 76: 263-270.

[26]   Goldstein FJ. Toxicity of cocaine. Compend Contin Educ Dent 1990; 11: 710-716.

[27]   Lee CY, Mohammedi H, Dixons RA. Medical and dental implications of cocaine abuse. J Oral Maxillofac Surg 1991; 49: 290-293.

[28]   Isaacs SO, Martin P, Willoughby JH. 'Crack' (an extra potent form of cocaine) abuse: a problem of the eighties. Oral Surg Oral Med Oral Pathol 1987; 63: 12-16.

[29]   Brewer JD, Meves A, Bostwick JM, Hamacher KL, Pittelkow MR. Cocaine abuse: dermatologic manifestations and therapeutic approaches. Journal of the American Academy of Dermatology 2008: 59(3): 483-487.

[30]   Maloney W. The Significance Of Illicit Drug Use To Dental Practice. WebmedCentral DENTISTRY, DRUG ABUSE 2010; 1(7): WMC00455.

[31]　Doyle AC. The Sign of Four. Spencer Blackett; London: 1890.

[32]　Musto DF. A Study in cocaine: Sherlock Holmes and Sigmund Freud. Journal of the American Medical Association 1968; 204(1): 27-32.

[33]　Pearce DN. Sherlock Holmes, Conan Doyle and cocaine. J Hist Neurosci 1994 Oct; 3(4): 227-232.

[34]　Maloney WJ. The Significance of cocaine use to dental practice. NY State Dent J 2010 Nov, 76 (6): 36-39.

[35]　Lange RA, Hillis LD. Cardiovascular complications of cocaine use. N Eng J Med 2001; 345(5): 351-358.

[36]　Brand HS, Gonggrijp S, Blanksma CJ. Cocaine and oral health. Brit Dent J 2008; 204: 365-369.

[37]　Cottrell DA, Mehra P, Malloy JC, Ghali GE. Midline palatal perforation. J Oral Maxillofac Surg 1999; 57: 990-995.

[38]　Talbott JF, Gorti GK, Kock RJ. Midfacial osteomyelitis in a chronic cocaine abuser: a case report. Ear Nose Throat J 2001; 80: 738-743.

[39]　Seyer BA, Grist W, Muller S. Aggressive destructive midfacial lesion from cocaine abuse. Oral Surg Oral Med Oral Pathol Oral Radiol Endod 2002; 94: 465-470.

[40]　Vilela RJ, Langford C, McCullagh L, Kass ES. Cocaine-induced oronasal fistulas with external nasal erosion but without palate involvement. Ear Nose Throat J 2002; 81: 562-563.

[41]　Brody SL, Slovis CM. Recognition and management of complications related to cocaine abuse. N Engl J Med. 1986 Dec 4: 315(23): 1495-1500.

[42]　Walsh SL, Stoops WW, Moody DE, Lin SN, Bigelow GE. Repeated dosing with oral cocaine in humans: assessment of direct effects, withdrawal, and pharmacokinetics. Exp Clin Psychopharmacol 2009 Aug; 17(4): 205-216.

[43]　Myers PJ. Drug abuse. 2009. Available at: www.mackenzie-media.com/chs/cmc/Publications/Dental/DrugAbuse.html.

[44]　Friedman DR, Wolfsthal SD. Cocaine-induced pseudovasculitis. Mayo Clinic Proc 2005; 80: 671-673.

[45]　Orriols R, Munoz X, Ferrer J, Huget P, Morell F. Cocaine-induced Ghurg-Strauss vasculitis. Eur Respir J 1996; 9: 175-177.

[46]　Noel B. Cocaine and arsenic-induced Raynaud's phenomenon. Clin Rheumatol 2002; 21: 343-344.

[47]　Balbir-Gurman A, Braun-Moscovici Y, Nahir AM. Cocaine-induced Raynaud's phenomenon and ischemic finger necrosis. Clin Rheumatol 2001; 20: 376-378.

[48]　Gertner E, Hamlar D. Necrotizing granulomatous vasculitis asscociated with cocaine use. J Rheumatol 2002; 29: 1795-1797.

[49]　Lu LK, High WA. Acute generalized exanthematous pustulosis caused by illicit street drugs? Arch Dermatol 2007; 143: 430-431.

[50]　Brust JC. Vasculitis owing to substance abuse. Neurol Clin 1997; 15: 945-957.

[51]　Chevalier X, Rostoker B, Larget-Piet B, Gherardi R. Schonlein-Henoch purpura with necrotizing vasculitis after cocaine snorting. Clin Nephrol 1995; 43: 348-349.

[52]　Hofbauer GF, Burg G, Nestle FO. Cocaine-related Stevens-Johnson syndrome. Dermatology 2000; 201: 258-260.

[53]　Marder VJ, Mellinghoff IK. Cocaine and Buerger disease: is there a pathogenic association? Arch Intern Med 2000; 160: 2057-2060.

[54]   Bozkurt AK. The role of cocaine in the etiology of Buerger disease is questionable. Arch Intern Med 2001; 161: 486.

[55]   Crandall CG, Vongpatanasin W, Victor RG. Mechanism of cocaine-induced hyperthermia in humans. Ann Intern Med 2002; 136: 785-791.

CHAPTER 30

Malaria: The Disease that Claimed the Life of the Boy Pharaoh

Abstract: King Tutankhamun was an Egyptian pharaoh who ruled from 1332 B.C. to 1332 B.C. His nearly intact tomb was discovered in 1922 by Howard Carter. Tutankhamun was probably the product of an incestuous relationship. This has led to much speculation concerning an inheritable genetic disorder being the cause of the young king's death. However, evidence points to malaria as being a more likely cause. Malaria is a potentially fatal mosquito-borne disease which is caused by a parasite. Illness and death from malaria can usually be prevented by the intervention of modern medicine.

Keywords: Amun, avascular necrosis, clubfoot, DNA, insecticide, malaria, mosquito, parasite, pharaoh, sickle-cell disorder, Soleb.

KING TUTANKHAMUN

Ancient Egypt has captured the collective imagination of people worldwide for thousands of years. The images of the pyramids and the Sphinx prompt us to wonder what it might have been to have lived during this fascinating period in the world's history. We have been provided glimpses into the ceremonies and traditions of Ancient Egypt through archaelogical studies. The life of Egypt's most famous ruler, King Tutankhamun, sheds some light on life in Ancient Egypt.

Tutankhamun, meaning "the living image of god Amun," was unconventional for his day. He introduced a new religion, shut down temples, banned other gods, and married his half-sister at the age of 12 [1]. During Tutankhamun's short reign- approximately 9 years- he repaired the temples of Amun, constructed his own tomb in the valley of the Kings, began the construction of the Temple of Karnak, and finished a pair of red granite lions at Soleb [2].

In 1907, Edward Russell Ayrton, a British archaeologist unearthed some artifacts in the Valley of the Kings. He subsequently announced that he had discovered the tomb of Tutankhamun and donated many of the artifacts to the New York

Metropolitan Museum of Art. Years later, a curator at the museum, Herbert Winlock, determined that these artifacts were merely objects from the boy pharaoh's funeral and embalming and not from the actual tomb. He theorized that the tomb had to be nearby. Winlock started a correspondence with Howard Carter. Carter subsequently started excavating the area in 1914 [3].

On November 4, 1922 the great British archaeologist Howard Carter found a few steps hidden beneath Egyptian soil. Finally, on February 16, 1923 Carter opened the sealed doorway which led directly to the burial chamber of Tutankhamun [4]. The New York Times called this day "the most extraordinary day in the history of Egyptian excavation [5]." His tomb was intact because its entrance had been hidden from tomb raiders by debris used in making a later tomb for King Ramses VI. In the tomb, there were so many objects- clothing, jewelry, hunting trophies, statues, and military items- that they still have not all been fully examined today [6-11]. In Carter's own words "... when, after about ten minutes' work, I had made a hole large enough to enable me to do so, I inserted an electric torch. An astonishing sight its light revealed, for there, within a yard of the doorway, stretching as far as one could see and blocking the entrance to the chamber, stood what to all appearances was a solid wall of gold ... It was, beyond any question, the sepulchral chamber in which we stood, for there, towering above us, was one of the great gilt shrines beneath which kings were laid. So enormous was this structure ... that it filled within a little the entire area of the chamber, a space of some two feet only separating it from the walls on all four sides, while its roof, with cornice top and torus moulding, reached almost to the ceiling ... [12]."

MALARIA

Malaria is a disease which is characterized by fever, headache, and vomiting. It is caused by a parasite and transmitted by infected mosquitoes. These parasites infect red blood cells after having multiplied in the liver [13]. One million individuals are killed worldwide by malaria each year [14]. Malaria is not common today in nations with a temperate climate such as the United States. However, it is still prevalent in tropical and subtropical nations.

A simple blood test can be used to diagnose malaria [15] which is extremely important as early diagnosis significantly increases the chances of survival.

Today there are certain anti-malarial drugs which protect non-immune individuals who travel to areas where malaria is an endemic disease. Chemoprophylaxis aims to reduce mortality and morbidity from malaria in young children and pregnant women in endemic areas. The unwanted effect, according to some studies, is the impairment of the development of natural acquired immunity [16].

Effective modern anti-malarial interventions include a prompt treatment with artemisinin- based combination therapies, insecticide spraying, and the use of insecticidal nets [16]. The world owes a great debt of gratitude to the many scientists who have dedicated their lives to work associated with malaria. In fact, four Nobel prizes have been awarded for this work- Sir Ronald Ross (1902), Charles Louis Alphonse Laveran (1907), Julius Wagner-Jauregg (1927), and Paul Hermann Muller (1948).

KING TUTANKHAMUN AND MALARIA

King Tutankhamun died around 1324 B.C. at the age of 19. The cause of his death has long been a source of speculation among historians and scientists alike. Some competing theories have been that he was murdered by his successor, Ay, or by some form of an accident [17]. Another theory is that Tutankhamun died of a genetic blood disease, sickle-cell disorder, as it occurs in 9 to 22 percent of individuals living in the Egyptian oases [18].

Recent evidence points to malaria and avascular necrosis being the cause of the young pharaoh's death [19]. Avascular necrosis is a disease in which tissue is destroyed or weakened due to a diminished blood supply to bone [20].

The case for malaria being the culprit certainly gains credence from the facts that, recently, DNA testing on the boy pharaoh's remains showed evidence of plasmodium falciparium which is the protozoan parasite that causes malaria in humans. Also supporting the malarial theory are the many canes and the veritable pharmacy found in his tomb [21].

Tutankhamun's left cheek and neck displayed areas of patchy skin changes. This could be the result of an inflamed mosquito bite or a mummification artifact [22]. Tutankhamun has also been shown through modern medical research and radiography to have had Kohler disease II, hypophalangism of the right foot and clubfoot on the left foot [23].

Many previous researchers were led astray in their search for the true cause of Tutankhamun's death by an x-ray which was taken back in the 1960's which revealed a hole in the pharaoh's skull. The research done by Hawass and colleagues demonstrates that the hole was probably made during the mummification process [23, 24].

REFERENCES

[1]   Marchant J. Ancient DNA: Curse of Pharaoh's DNA. Nature 472, 404-406 (2011).
[2]   BBC. Tutankhamun (1336 BC-1327 BC). Accessed on November 2, 2013. Available at: http://www.bbc.co.uk/history/historic_figures?tutankhamun.shtml.
[3]   The New York Times. Howard Carter, 64, Egyptologist, Dies. March 3, 1939.
[4]   Covington R. King Tut: the Pharaoh Returned. Smithsonian Magazine. June 2005.
[5]   The New York Times. Tut-ankh-Amen's Inner Tomb is Opened Revealing Undreamed of Splendors still Untouched after 3,400 years. February 16, 1923.
[6]   Encyclopedia of World Biography. Tutankhamen Biography. Accessed on October 29, 2013. Available at: www.notablebiographies.com/Tu-We/Tutankhamen.htm/#b.
[7]   Brier B. The Murder of Tutankhamen: a True Story. New York: Putnam, 1998.
[8]   Carter H and Mace AC. The Tomb of Tut-ankh-amen. New York: Cooper Square Publishers, 1963.
[9]   Desroches-Noblecourt C. Tutankhamen: Life and Death of a Pharaoh. Garden City, NY: Doubleday, 1965.
[10]   El Mahdy C. Tutankhamen: The Life and Death of the Boy-King. New York: St. Martin's Press, 2000.
[11]   James TGH. Tutankhamun. Vercelli, Italy: Friedman/Fairfax Publishers, 2000.
[12]   Reeves N. The Complete Tutankhamun: The King, the Tomb, the Royal Treasure (London: Thames and Hudson Ltd., 1990) 79.
[13]   World Health Organization. Malaria. Accessed on November 4, 2013. Available at: http://www.who.int/topics/malaria/en/
[14]   Mayo Clinic. Malaria. Accessed on November 2, 2013. Available at: http://www.mayoclinic.com/health/malaria/DS00475.
[15]   MedlinePlus. Malaria. Accessed on November 1, 2013. Available at: http://www.nlm.nih.gov/medlineplus/malaria.html.
[16]   Greenwood B. The Use of anti-malarial drugs to prevent malaria in the population of malaria-endemic areas. Journal of Tropical Medicine and Hygiene January 2004; 7(1): 1-7.

[17]   KTVU. King Tut Bio. Accessed on November 2, 2013. Available at: http://www.ktvu.com/news/news/king-tut-bio/wkzbh/.

[18]   Wuyts A. The Independent. King Tut died from sickle- cell disease, not malaria; June 25, 2000.

[19]   Cheng Q, Cloonan N, Fischer K, *et al*. Stevor and rif are Plasmodium falciparum multicopy gene families which potentially encode variant antigens. Mol Biochem Parasitol. 1998; 97(1-2): 161-176.

[20]   Wilford JN. Malaria is a likely killer in King Tut's post mortem. New York Times. February 16, 2010.

[21]   Alleyae R. the Guardian. king Tut died of malaria and bone condition, says new research. February 16, 2010.

[22]   Leek F. The Human remains from the tomb of Tutankhamen. Oxford, UK: Tutankhamun Tomb Series V; 1972.

[23]   Hawass Z, Gady Z, Ismail S, Khairat R, Fathalla D, Hasan N, Ahmed A, Elleithy H, Ball M, Gaballah F, Wassef S, Fateen M, Selim A, Zink A, Carsten. Ancestry and patholgy in King Tutankhamun's family. JAMA 2010, 303(7): 638-647.

[24]   Willingham V. Malaria, genetic diseases plagued King Tut. Accessed on November 3, 2013. Available at: http://www.cnn.com/2010/HEALTH/02/16/king.tut.malaria/.

CHAPTER 31

George Washington's Teeth or, the Lack Thereof

Abstract: Myths and legends surround every aspect of the life of George Washington. Prominent among the Washingtonian myths is that he had wooden teeth. Washington never had teeth made of wood. They were the most modern dentures of the time. They were also very uncomfortable and painful. Millions of individuals worldwide, like Washington, have lost some or all of their natural teeth. There are various causes for tooth loss. There are also multiple treatment options to replace the missing teeth. Such options include dentures, dental implants, and cemented dental bridges.

Keywords: Cemented dental bridges, complete dentures, fluoride, Marshalsea Prison, mouthrinses, myths, partial dentures, Pope's Creek, surveyor, wooden teeth.

GEORGE WASHINGTON

It was March of 1793 somewhere in the North Atlantic. American born portrait artist Gilbert Stuart was sailing from London to the new nation. In addition to being a brilliant portrait artist, Stuart was a debtor having been imprisoned in Dublin's Marshalsea Prison. Stuart was a disheveled, talkative, impulsive, restless, alcoholic, harried spendthrift. He was coming back to the land of his birth to make his fortune and pay his creditors by painting the portrait of America's first president, George Washington, whom he had never met. In fact Washington didn't even know that Stuart existed.

The great historian and biographer Ron Chernow used the term "stalked" to describe Stuart's approach to meeting Washington's friend and Chief Justice John Jay [1]. John Jay agreed to have Stuart produce a portrait of himself. Stuart's portrait of John Jay has been described as being majestic and brilliant [1]. In return, Jay gave Stuart a letter of introduction to the new president.

By contrast, Washington was a regal 6 foot 2 inch, 175 pound living icon. Washington consciously attempted to subdue and conceal any of his emotions throughout his life. During one of Washington's first sittings with Stuart, Stuart attempted to uncover the human side of Washington hidden below the stone-cold exterior. Stuart later told friends that he never saw physical characteristics similar to Washington in any of his previous subjects. He saw an almost savage fire hidden in Washington's eyes.

During the sitting, Stuart told Washington that he should forget that he is the great General Washington and Stuart only a painter. Washington quickly replied that Stuart should never forget neither who Washington is nor who Stuart the painter is.

Nonetheless, Stuart was an artistic genius and was able to draw out the fire in Washington's soul which usually lay hidden beneath Washington's frozen countenance. The unlikely pairing of Washington and Stuart would produce a series of portraits. The most famous of these paintings, known as The Athenaeum, is portrayed on the dollar bill of the United States. Another of Stuart's portraits of Washington hung in the White House and was heroically saved from certain desecration by the British during the War of 1812 as Dolley Madison insisted on saving the portrait while abandoning her and her husband's personal belongings.

The life of the majestic Washington began at his father's plantation on Pope's Creek in Westmoreland County, Virginia on February 22, 1732. George's father, Augustine, died when George was eleven years ago. George attended school around his home for the next few years until his formal education ended at the age of fifteen. Young George was an adventurous teenager and desired to join the British Navy but his mother refused to give him permission so George had to settle for accompanying George William Fairfax, a surveyor, into the Virginia wilderness. By the time George was seventeen years old he had received an appointment as the county surveyor for Culpeper County [2]. By the time George was 21, he owned more than 1,500 acres all purchased with his own earnings.

Washington's older brother, Lawrence, died during this period and bequeathed upon his younger sibling his Mount Vernon estate and requested that he replace his office as adjutant general of the colony [3]. By 1754 Washington was a colonel in the French and Indian War. His military reputation and prowess would grow over the next two decades. In 1775, Washington was appointed to a position that he neither sought nor would be paid for- Commander-in-Chief of the Continental Army [3].

After a tumultuous six years, Washington accepted the surrender of Lord General Cornwallis at Yorktown, Virginia on October 19, 1781. Cornwallis was conspicuously absent that afternoon from the surrender ceremonies as he said he felt ill. Considering the events of the day, his excuse seems plausible. Cornwallis' substitute, General O'Hara, attempted to surrender to Comte de Rochambeau who, in turn, directed him to General Washington [4].

The new nation now needed a leader. The obvious choice was Washington due to his intelligence and humble spirit. The fact that Washington had no children, particularly no sons, made the choice even easier. After serving his nation as the first president, Washington yearned to retire to his beautiful estate. He got his wish, albeit for only three years as he died of a throat infection on December 14, 1799 [5].

Fisher Ames wrote a eulogy dated February 8, 1800. He described Washington as being one of "that small number ... who were no less distinguished for the elevation of their virtues than the luster of their talents ... who were born, and who acted through life as if they were born, not for themselves, but for their country and the whole human race" [6].

EDENTULISM

Edentulism is a dental term which refers to an individual having lost some or all of their teeth. An individual having lost some of their teeth is referred to as being partial edentulous while complete edentulism refers to an individual having lost all of their natural teeth.

Fortunately, dentistry has made incredible strides since the primitive days of Washington. An individual who has lost some or all of their natural teeth has many options for replacing these teeth and living a normal, healthy and comfortable life. The first step in replacing the missing teeth, in the case of partial edentulism, is for the patient's dentist to identify the reason behind the patient's loss of teeth. If the reason is tooth decay, all remaining decay should be first removed in the remaining teeth. The dentist most also identify the risk factors which are present for tooth decay in the patient. Sometimes a patient who has tooth decay might be eating foods which promote dental caries. In such a case the dentist should analyze the patient's diet and discuss possible alterations to the diet with the patient. An example of this would be the elimination of soft drinks which have a high sugar content. The dentist will also instruct the patient in proper oral hygiene techniques and might recommend various fluoride- containing toothpastes or mouthrinses. It is also imperative that the patient be placed on a proper dental recall schedule for cleanings and oral examinations in consideration of the patient's risk for tooth decay and periodontal disease.

DENTURES

There are two main types of dentures- partial dentures and complete dentures.

Partial dentures, like complete dentures, are removable. That means that they are not cemented in the individual's mouth. Partial dentures are made out of a variety of materials. They get their retention from both the surrounding teeth and the natural oral structures.

Complete dentures are for individuals who have no remaining teeth on either the upper or lower arches, or both. Complete dentures obtain their retention from the anatomic structures of the mouth. For added retention, particularly in the lower arch, implants are commonly placed. This results in an implant-supported denture.

CEMENTED BRIDGES

Cemented bridges are an option for replacing one or more missing teeth. Some of the advantages of a cemented bridge are that it is non-removable, very lifelike, and improves masticatory function.

Cemented bridges require the dentist to shape the teeth on either side of the missing tooth or teeth. These teeth are shaped into very specific dimensions which will eventually become the anchors for the final bridge.

After the dentist is satisfied that the preparations of the abutment teeth are proper, an impression is made of the arch of teeth where the bridge is being constructed. Another impression is made of the opposing arch so that the proper occlusion or bite can be achieved.

A great amount of work is done in constructing the fixed bridge by a commercial dental laboratory. They perform various tasks in constructing a patient's bridge. This includes waxing copings which they subsequently cast into the metal understructure of the final bridge. Porcelain is then applied to the metal portion of the bridge in the proper shade to match the patient's other teeth. Sometimes today, the entire bridge can be made out of ceramics in order to have a more esthetic result. This is dependent upon various technical details which the dentist must analyze.

Once the dentist has the finished bridge back from the laboratory, he or she will try-in the bridge to ensure a proper fit and patient satisfaction. After everyone is satisfied with the quality of the bridge the dentist is able to cement the final fixed prosthesis.

DENTAL IMPLANTS

Dental implants are an excellent option for replacing a single tooth or multiple teeth. The key to the success of dental implants is a process known as osseointegration. Osseointegration refers to the process by which the patient's bone grows into direct contact with the titanium metal of the implant which has been placed into the patient's upper or lower jaw. For osseointegration to occur there can be no soft tissue between the bone and the implant.

Modern dental implantology allows for the replacement of one or more teeth. A trained dental professional surgically places the implant fixture into the bone. An abutment needs to be placed onto the fixture which will allow for a permanent prosthesis or tooth replacement to be provided to the patient.

The most important aspect of the entire implant process is for the dentist to develop a proper treatment plan. Certain diagnostic impressions need to be made as well as various X-rays.

For implants that will replace a single tooth, the dentist must be concerned that adequate space is available between the adjacent teeth. Another concern is that the ridge of bone is of a sufficient diameter.

Sometimes for implants on the maxillary or upper arch, the sinus is located in a manner whereby sinus augmentation or a sinus lift would be required to ensure that the implant will have an adequate length.

Implants for single teeth have the great positive quality of not necessitating the preparation and, therefore, reduction of tooth structure as do cemented bridges. Whenever possible, it is advisable to preserve healthy tooth structure.

WASHINGTON'S TEETH

Looking skyward towards the dome of the United States Capitol Building in Washington, D.C. one will view a 4,664 square foot fresco by Constantino Brumidi. The fresco is named 'The Apotheosis of Washington'. It was painted over a period of 11 months around 1864. Apotheosis is a word which refers to the process of making a human being into a god. This is exactly what happened to Washington in the years following his death. His supporters and admirers went on a vigorous campaign to make the first president of the United States into a form of a deity. Washington was certainly revered in life but, in death, he would sit on an exalted throne surrounded by his fellow immortals such as Ceres, Vulcan, Neptune, and Mercury and flanked by the goddess Victoria to his left and the goddess Liberty to his right.

Brumidi's fresco was merely one aspect of the deification of Washington. Many legends were made up about Washington. Many of these legends attempted to portray Washington's impeccable moral character or his inner fortitude. One such legend was that Washington had wooden teeth. This would dramatize the stoic qualities of Washington. The exact origin of this legend remains unclear but what probably gave some credence to this legend was that the ivory teeth used by Washington's dentist, John Greenwood, probably stained over time giving the teeth a wooden, dark appearance [7]. Washington even addressed this appearance in a 1798 letter to Greenwood, "the sett you sent me from Philadelphia... was very black ... Port wine being very sower takes off all the polish." [8]

A letter dated May 29, 1781 from Washington to Dr. Baker gives some insight to the amount of thought and effort that Washington was forced to dedicate to his teeth, or more appropriately, to the lack thereof. Washington wrote, "New Windsor May 29, 1781 / Sir, A day or two ago I requested / Col. Harrison to apply to you for a pair/ of Pincers to fasten the wire of my teeth. -- I hope / you furnished him with them.-- I now wish/ you would send me one of your scrapers / as my teeth stand in need of cleaning, and / I have little prospect of being in Philadelph. / soon.-- It will come very safe by the Post-- / & in return, the money shall be sent so soon as/ I know the cost of it.-- / I am Sir / Y Very H Serv [Your Very Humble Servant] / G. Washington [9]."

Washington's dental troubles began when he was only 21 years-old. Washington suffered from constant dental pain as a result of dental infections, abscesses, periodontal issues, and poorly fitting dentures (Table **12**). By the time he took the presidential oath of office he only had one tooth in his mouth and was wearing his first set of full dentures which were made for him by John Greenwood. The upper denture had teeth made from hippopotamus ivory. The lower consisted of eight human teeth with gold pivots screwed into the base. These teeth made life very unpleasant and painful [10-19].

It is thought that Washington did not give a speech at his second presidential inauguration because of pain and discomfort arising from his dental issues [10]. Washington was only able to eat soft foods towards the end of his life.

Table 12. **Recognized Dental Specialties**

-Dental Public Health (promotes dental health through community efforts)
-Periodontics (gingiva and surrounding bone)
-Oral and Maxillofacial Surgery (extractions)
-Oral and Maxillofacial Pathology (oral diseases)
-Endodontics (root canals)
-Pediatric dentistry (children's dentistry)
-Prosthodontics (crowns, dentures)
-Oral and Maxillofacial Radiology (x-rays)
-Orthodontics and Dentofacial Orthopedics (braces)

REFERENCES

[1]   Chernow R. Washington: a life. 2010; The Penguin Press: USA.

[2]   George Washington's Mount Vernon. Biography of George Washington. Accessed on October 1, 2013. Available at: http://www.mountvernon.org/georgewashington.

[3]   XRoads. Toward Fact: a biography. Accessed on October 1, 2013. Available at: http://xroads.virginia.edu/-cap/gw/gwbio.html.

[4]   Eyewitness To History. Yorktown. Accessed on: October 1, 2013. Available at: http://www.eyewitnesstohistory.com/yorktown.htm.

[5]   The White House. George Washington. Accessed on October 1, 2013. Available at: http://www.whitehouse.gov/about/presidents/georgewashington.

[6]   Works of Fisher Ames, ed. William B. Allen, Volume I (Indianapolis: Liberty Classics, 1983), 519-538.

[7]   John Greenwood to George Washington, New York, 28 December 1789, in ed. Dorothy Twohig, The Papers of George Washington. Retirement Series, Vol. 3 (Charlottesville: University of Virginia Press, 1988): 289.

[8]   George Washington's Mount Vernon. Wooden teeth myth. Accessed on October 11, 2013 Available at: http://www.Wooden%20Teeth%20Myth%20%7C%20George %20Washington's%20Mount%20Vernon.com.

[9]   University of Michigan Letter from George Washington to Dr.Baker. May 20, 1781.

[10]   Glover B. George Washington- a dental victim. Accessed on October 13, 2013. Available at: http://www.americanrevolution.org.dental.html

[11]   Callcott, GH. A History of the University of Maryland., Maryland Historical Society, Baltimore, MD.

[12]   Hillam C. Ed. for Lindsay Society for History of Dentistry 1990. Roots of Dentistry pub. by British Dental Assoc.

[13]   Hoffman-Axthelm, W. Translated by H. M. Koehler. History of Dentistry. Quintessence Pub. Co. 1981.

[14]   Klatell, Jack DDS. Kaplan, Andrew DMD, Williams, Gray, Jr. illus: Caroline Meinstein. The Mount Sinai medical Center- Family Guide to Dental Health. MacMillan Publ. Co. 1991.

[15]   The Dr. Samuel D. Harris Mational Museum of Dentistry, Baltimore, MD.

[16]   Prinz H. Dental Chronology: A record of the more important events in the evolution of dentistry. Lea & Fehiger, Philadelphia, PA.

[17]   Ring ME. Dentistry: An Illustrated History. Henry N. Abrams, Inc., C.V. Mosby Co. 1985.

[18]   Stier CJ. papers, Baron Henry deWitte's Archives, Antwerp.

[19]   Weinberger, BW. Introduction to History of Dentistry in America Vol. I & II. C.V. Mosby Co. 1948.

CHAPTER 32

Rip van Winkle Syndrome: a Medical Phenomenon from the Peaks of the Hudson Valley

Abstract: Washington Irving was an American author who wrote a short story about a man who fell asleep for twenty years and then suddenly awoke to find that the world had changed dramatically during his odd slumber. This eponymous literary character has given his name to a condition known in the medical literature as Kleine-Levin Syndrome. Rip Van Winkle Syndrome refers to this disorder which is found mainly in adolescent boys and is characterized by hypersomnolence. There is no cure for this syndrome. However, like Rip van Winkle's slumber, the disorder suddenly disappears after a period of years.

Keywords: Adolescent, antiepileptic mood stabilizer, apathy, Catskills, childlike behavior, confusion, hypersexuality, Kleine-Levin Syndrome, lethargy, modanafil.

WASHINGTON IRVING

On April 3, 1783 Washington Irving was born in New York City. He was named after the hero of America's revolution, George Washington. Irving even attended the presidential inauguration of Washington in 1789 in lower Manhattan. He became a prolific writer, a champion of international copyright law, and the United States ambassador to Spain. He would be best remembered for two of his short stories, 'Rip Van Winkle' and 'The Legend of Sleepy Hollow'. Both of these stories recant the charms, legends, and bucolic traditions of life in the late eighteenth century Hudson Valley. The Hudson Valley is a special location lying just north of New York City and extending past the state capital in Albany. The region is dominated by beautiful mountains and the mighty river which bears the name of the great explorer, Hendrick Hudson, who navigated its currents in his Half Moon.

In 1815, Irving travelled to London to work for his brothers in their business venture. This business soon failed and Irving looked towards writing as a means to support himself. His two great works were published in 1819 as a collection of short stories and essays in 'The Sketch Book' [1].

Washington continued to write for the remainder of his life and became known as America's first man of letters. He published, in the 1830's, 'Astoria', 'Adventures of Captain Bonneville, USA' and 'The Far West'.

There has been much scholarly debate over the past two centuries concerning both the quality and meaning of his literary work. Some feel that his work, particularly 'The Legend of Sleepy Hollow', reveals Irving's fear of male disempowerment. Others feel that his work contains too many European analogies and references and possess too many reservations about the nascent country to be truly representative of a distinctive American nationalistic style [1-3]. Nonetheless, I believe that Irving's work was truly emblematic of the feelings of the new nation which were, at times, ambivalent. The settlers in Irving's Hudson Valley had European roots which could not be denied. They brought their customs to the region and combined them with new traditions and customs of the region. That was the essence of the early days of the nation and Irving captured those feelings masterfully.

People still enjoy and celebrate the works of Irving today in the Hudson Valley. In beautiful Westchester County visitors explore Irving's magnificent home, Sunnyside. In another Westchester village, not coincidentally named Sleepy Hollow, Washington Irving is buried in the cemetery which lies next to the Old Dutch Church where the infamous Headless Horseman used to ride on moonlit gallops.

RIP VAN WINKLE

Washington Irving published 'Rip van Winkle' as a short story in 1819 as part of a collection entitled 'The Sketch Book of Geoffrey Crayon, Gent'. The story is set in a very old village at the foot of the beautiful and magical Catskill Mountains. The Catskill region is located in New York state approximately 70 miles north of New York City. This region had many early Dutch settlers.

The reader is told that Rip van Winkle [5] was a kind and gentle man who would rather talk to his friends and neighbors all day rather than labor in his own fields. He is married to Dame van Winkle who is not hesitant to insult her simple husband. In order to escape his wife, he would sit on a bench outside the inn of Nicholaus Vedder and trade sleepy stories about nothing with other men.

One day Rip travelled to a very high point in the mountain and sat down to rest. After some time he was approached by an odd-looking man dressed in old-fashioned Dutch clothes. Rip helped this man carry a keg to an even higher point on the mountain. There were other similarly odd men at their destination. These men were bowling and offered Rip a very good-tasting drink. Rip had another drink and another and another and ...

Rip awakes in the morning light. He was completely confused because his gun had become old and rusty. The surrounding area looked unfamiliar and his dog was nowhere to be found. Things became stranger yet when he arrived in his village and he didn't see one familiar face. Even the picture in his favorite inn had been changed. The portrait of Great Britain's King George III had been replaced with one of someone known as George Washington. Subsequently, he learned that Nicholaus Vedder had been dead for many years and he couldn't find his own family.

Rip was then approached by a woman who looked vaguely familiar to him. She told him that her father went for a walk one day twenty years ago and never returned. Rip soon realized that this woman was his daughter. Despite his fear, he was delighted to hear that his wife, Dame van Winkle, had passed away.

The village's oldest resident, Peter Vanderdonk, identified Rip. Peter went on to state that he had heard tales in the magical Catskills of the ghosts of the great explorer of the region, Hendrick Hudson, and his men reappearing every twenty years to bowl and to guard the region.

Rip went on to live the rest of his life in idle peace and happiness with his daughter and her farmer husband.

KLEINE-LEVIN SYNDROME

The Rip van Winkle Syndrome is known in medical terminology as Kleine-Levin Syndrome (KLS). KLS affects mainly adolescents and is a rare and complex neurological disorder. Individuals with KLS experience periods of excessive amounts of sleep and altered behavior. Initial stages of an episode of KLS can be characterized by the individual becoming progressively drowsy and sleeping for much of the duration of both the day and night. The individual becomes lethargic, childlike, disoriented, confused, and apathetic. They usually also experience a hypersensitivity to both noise and light and their visual acumen is poor. Some individuals experiencing an episode of KLS also experience food cravings and uninhibited hypersexuality [6] (Table **13**).

Table 13.   Signs and Symptoms of Kleine-Levin Syndrome

-childlike demeanor
-hypersomnolence
-apathy
-lethargy
-confusion
-objects out of focus
-compulsive hyperphagia
-uninhibited hypersexuality

KLS is an episodic disorder. Arnulf *et al.* state that, in two-thirds of observed patients, there was an infection at the onset of the disease [7]. Treatment of KLS is far from predictable. Amphetamine stimulants, lithium, and antiepileptic mood stabilizers have all been used in treating the disease with varying degrees of success [8]. Modafinil has been shown to be useful in reducing the duration of the episode of symptomologies while no treatment or medication of any kind has been demonstrated to be effective in preventing the recurrence of an episode of KLS [8]. The syndrome eventually disappears spontaneously [9] after a period of 4-8 years.

REFERENCES

[1]   Washington Irving. (2013). The Biography Channel website. Accessed on October 3, 2013. Available at: http://www.biography.com/people/washington-irving-9350087.

[2]   Paul R. "Chapter 3: Washington Irving." PAL: Perspectives in American Litera-ture- A Research and reference Guide, WWW URL: http://web.csustan.edu/ english/reub en/pal/chap3/irving.html. Accessed on October 3, 2013.

[3]   Bylington, J. Introduction. Nineteenth Century Literature Criticism. Michigan: Gale Group, 200: 98, 216-303.

[4]   Cracroft R. Washington Irving: the western works. Boise: Boise State University, 1974.

[5]   The Complete works of Washington Irving. (Rust, *et al.*, editors). 30 vols. (University of Wisconsin/ Twayne, 1969-1986).

[6]   Kleine-Levin Syndrome Foundation. What is Kleine-Levin Syndrome? Accessed on October 2, 2013. Available at: http://klsfoundation.org/kleine/levin/info/ what_is_kleine_le vin_syndrome.

[7]   Arnulf I, Zeitzer JM, Farber N, Mignot E. Kleine-Levin Syndrome: a systematic review of 186 cases in the literature. Brain 2005 Dec; 128 (Pt 12): 2763- 2776. Epub 2005 Oct 17.

[8]   Huang YS, Lakki SC, Guilleminault C. Kleine-Levin Syndrome: current status. Med Clin North Am. 2010 May; 94(3): 557-562.

[9]   Pearce JM. Kleine-Levin syndrome: history and brief review. Eur Neurol 2008; 60(4): 212-214 Epub 2008 Jul 30.

CHAPTER 33

The Deafness of Beethoven

Abstract: Ludwig van Beethoven was the greatest musical composer that the world has ever known. In a tragic twist of irony, the creator of the most beloved musical compositions became deaf in the prime of his life and career. Many historians have attempted to determine the cause of this deafness. The most logical diagnosis is Paget's disease. Paget's disease is a chronic metabolic disorder that is characterized by the abnormal formation and resorption of bone. The disease most likely caused Beethoven's deafness by compressing his eighth cranial nerve.

Keywords: Beethoven, deafness, ear malformation, hearing loss, jaundice, Mozart, Napoleon, otitis media, Paget's disease, premature birth, presbyacusis, Salieri, the Eroica Symphony.

BEETHOVEN

Ludwig van Beethoven was born on December 16 or 17, 1770 in Bonn, Germany to a father who was a musician and could be described as an alcoholic. Beethoven's mother, Maria Magdalena van Beethoven, was described by her contemporaries as being a kind, gently and loving lady. Beethoven called his mother "his best friend" [1]. Beethoven's father attempted to teach him music but, unfortunately, he wasn't much of either a teacher or a musician himself. However, he desperately wanted to create a musical giant in his son. He introduced his son to the public at age 7 when, on March 26, 1778, the young child gave his first public performance at Cologne.

The father was fortunately intelligent enough to realize that his talented young son needed a much better musical teacher and mentor than himself. Gottlob Neefe tutored the youth in organ and composition as well as the works of the great philosophers. At the age of 12 Beethoven published his first work, 9 Variations in C Minor for piano on a march by Earnst Christoph Dressler.

In 1787 Beethoven was sent to Vienna to study under Mozart. After auditioning for the great composer, Mozart stated "Keep your eyes on him; some day he will give the world something to talk about." Unfortunately, after only a few weeks of study Beethoven received word that his mother had fallen ill. He returned home immediately to be with his gravely ill mother who died seven months later. This scarred Beethoven and caused him to enter a state of depression which lasted several years.

When the Holy Roman Emperor Joseph II died in 1790, Beethoven was asked to compose a musical memorial. Beethoven was 19 years old. No composition in honor of the Holy Roman Emperor was ever performed and everyone assumed that the young Beethoven had been incapable of producing the work. Over a century later Johannes Brahms discovered a composition entitled 'Cantata on the Death of Emperor Joseph II.' Brahms called it "beautiful and noble". It is now considered to be Beethoven's earliest masterpiece [2].

In 1792, Beethoven started studying piano with Joseph Haydn, vocal composition with Antonio Salieri and counterpoint with Johann Albrechtsberger. Beethoven would subsequently compose many pieces and reach his musical maturity over the next period of years.

In 1804, Beethoven debuted his Symphony No. 3 in honor of Napoleon who had only weeks before proclaimed himself Emperor of France. At first, Beethoven admired and identified with Napoleon. He would later become disillusioned with Napoleon and changed the name of the symphony to the Eroica Symphony.

Beethoven fought with everyone he was involved with throughout his adult life. These individuals included his brothers, patrons, pupils, housekeepers, and publishers. Beethoven never married and had no children but, was madly in love with a married woman. He referred to Antonie Brentano, in an undelivered letter, as "my Immortal Beloved".

Beethoven's Ninth and final symphony contains a choral finale with four vocal soloists and a chorus singing the words of Friedrich Schiller's poem "Ode to Joy". This is considered to be the most famous piece of music in history [2].

Beethoven passed away on March 26, 1827 at the age of 56 of post-hepatic cirrhosis of the liver.

DEAFNESS

There are a multitude of causes of deafness. Some of these causes result in congenital deafness while others cause individuals to become progressively more deaf as they age [3].

Congenital deafness may be due to a genetic disease such as Waardenburg Syndrome or may be the result of a certain abnormal physical trait such as an ear malformation. The health of the pregnant mother also can result in hearing loss of the newborn. Certain ototoxic drugs taken by the mother may result in deafness as well if the mother has rubella, syphilis or cytomegalovirus.

A premature birth, lack of oxygen, jaundice, or head trauma to the infant at birth have the potential for hearing loss.

An inflammation in the middle ear known as otitis media can damage the eardrum and middle ear. These structures function in the transmission of sound thus potentially resulting in hearing loss.

Progressive hearing loss in older people is known as terminal presbyacusis. It results from the nerve cells in the inner ear starting to degenerate. These nerve cells are responsible for converting sounds into nervous impulses.

There are various ototoxic drugs. These drugs damage the hair cells which convert sounds into nervous impulses either in the inner ear and/or to the auditory nerve. Examples of ototoxic drugs are streptomycin, quinine, and chloroquine.

Tinnitus is a ringing sound in the ear which could be triggered by noise-induced hearing loss, excess wax in the ear canal, medications, ear or sinus infections, acoustic nerve tumors and cardiovascular diseases [3].

Hearing loss can adversely affect one's quality of life. Older individuals might suffer from depression or anxiety as a result of the hearing loss. They might also, incorrectly, feel that others are angry with them [4]. It is imperative that individuals who are experiencing the initial stages of hearing loss seek medical attention.

One interesting recent study shows that progesterone, a sex hormone, has a negative effect on the hearing of older women and aging mice while estrogen might have a positive influence. This could eventually lead to biomedical interventions to modulate or prevent age-related hearing loss [5].

BEETHOVEN'S DEAFNESS

By the age of 28 Beethoven began to lose his hearing. There has been much speculation concerning the cause of Beethoven's deafness. The most reasonable post- mortem diagnosis is Paget's disease. The disease process most likely compressed his eighth cranial nerve resulting in the loss of hearing.

Beethoven developed many symptoms which are consistent with a diagnosis of Paget's disease. These include an enlarging head, a prominent forehead, a large jaw, and a protruding chin [6].

In 1877, Sir James Paget first described Paget disease of bone. He referred to it as osteitis deformans. It is a chronic metabolic disease where there is abnormal formation and resorption of bone. The major characteristic of the disease is enlargement of the bone. Bone pain, deafness, bowing of the legs, dizziness, weakness, and loss of hearing are all complications of the disease [7].

Beethoven's loss of hearing progressed through the years starting with severe tinnitus followed by a loss of higher frequencies. During his adult life Beethoven would suffer from other maladies including frequent infections, colitis, chronic hepatitis, chronic pancreatitis, rheumatism, and splenomegaly [8-10].

During the initial stage of his hearing loss, Beethoven could hear certain high tones and loud speech. He adapted well to his hearing loss. Beethoven's Graf piano had an added amplification apparatus and he used a sound conductor to hear himself play at the keyboard until 1826. He also used an ear trumpet to hear certain people's speech until the same year [11]. In the last years of his life, Beethoven used 'conversation books' to communicate with visitors and friends [12].

On March 27, 1827 Karl Rokitansky performed an autopsy on the remains of the great composer. He identified conditions which are consistent with a diagnosis of Paget's disease. These include shriveled auditory nerves and a uniformly dense skull vault. He concluded that Beethoven had died as a result of an alcoholic liver disease [6].

REFERENCES

[1]   Biography. Ludwig van Beethoven's biography. Available at: http://www.lvbeethoven. com/Bio/BiographyLudwig.html. Accessed on: September 13, 2013.

[2]   Bio.true story. Ludwig van Beethoven. Accessed on September 11, 2013. Available at: http://www.biography.com/people/ludwig-van-beethoven-9204862?page=5.

[3]   CBM. CBM International Causes of Deafness. Accessed on7/11/13.Available at: http://www.cbm.org/causes-of-deafness-251493.php.

[4]   Mayo   Clinic.   Hearing   Loss.   Accessed   on   6/3/13.Available   at: http:// www.mayoclinic.com/health/hearing-loss/DS001721DSECTION=complications

[5]   Frisina RD, Frisina DR. Physiological and neurobiological bases of age-related hearing loss: biotherapeutic implications. Am J Audiol 2013 Sep 9 [Epub ahead of print].

[6]   Wolf P. Creativity and chronic disease Ludwig van Beethoven (1770-1827). West J Med 2001; 175(5): 298.

[7]   Sedano HO. Paget disease of bone. Accessed on May 25, 2013. Available at: www.dent.ucla.edu/pic/visitors/pdb/page1.html.

[8]   Larkin E. Beethoven's illness: a likely diagnosis. Proc Roy Soc Med 1971; 64: 493-500.

[9]   Naiken VS. Did Beethoven have Paget's disease of bone? Ann Intern Med 1971; 74: 995-999.

[10]   McCabe GE. Beethoven's deafness. Ann Otol 1958; 67: 192-206.

[11]   Mai FM. Diagnosing genius: the life and death of Beethoven. 2007; McGill-Queen's University.

[12]   Cooper M. Ludwig van Beethoven. Music Critic, The London Telegraph London EC4.

INDEX

A

S

T

www.ingramcontent.com/pod-product-compliance
Lightning Source LLC
Chambersburg PA
CBHW050841220326
41598CB00006B/420